D0303320

Self-Assessment Colour Review of

Renal Medicine

T

DATE OF RETURN
UNLESS RECALLED BY LIBRARY

2 3 JAN 2007	– 2 OCT 2009
1 8 APR 2007	10/2/11
1 1 MAY 2007	2 5 MAY 2011
2 1 MAY 2007	28/10/14
2 1 MAY 2007	
3 0 MAY 2007	
CANCEL 2007	
CANCEL 2007	
– 8 APR 2008	
1 5 APR 2008	

CANCEL CANCEL CANCEL

PLEASE TAKE GOOD CARE OF THIS BOOK

UNIVERSITY OF
SHEFFIELD
LIBRARY

Self-Assessment Colour Review of Renal Medicine
Timothy H.J. Goodship and Bradley J. Maroni
ISBN: 1–874545–42–1

This edition reissued in 2003

Copyright © 1997, 2003 Manson Publishing Ltd

All rights reserved. No part of this publication may be reproduced, stored in a
retrieval system or transmitted in any form or by any means without the written
permission of the copyright holder or in accordance with the provisions of the
Copyright Act 1956 (as amended), or under the terms of any licence permitting
limited copying issued by the Copyright Licensing Agency, 33–34 Alfred Place,
London WC1E 7DP, UK.

Any person who does any unauthorized act in relation to this publication may be
liable to criminal prosecution and civil claims for damages.

A CIP catalogue record for this book is available from the British Library.

For full details of all Manson Publishing Ltd titles please write to:
Manson Publishing Ltd, 73 Corringham Road, London NW11 7DL, UK.

Tel: +44(0)20 8905 5150
Fax: +44(0)20 8201 9233

Email: manson@man-pub.demon.co.uk
Website: www.manson-publishing.co.uk

Printed and bound in Spain and the United Kingdom

Preface

For many physicians renal medicine is a daunting subject, but because of the pivotal role of the kidneys in maintaining the *milieu intérieur* its importance cannot be underestimated. Questions pertaining to renal medicine are regularly found in postgraduate medical examinations such as the Membership of the Royal College of Physicians of the United Kingdom and the Boards examinations of the United States. This book is therefore intended primarily for doctors in training who are approaching such examinations, but will also provide an up-to-date review for all clinicians. By providing detailed answers, we hope that not only will knowledge be tested, but also increased.

The questions intentionally cover a broad range of renal medicine, including physiology, fluid and electrolyte balance, clinical nephrology, haemodialysis, peritoneal dialysis and transplantation. We have included questions which involve the interpretation of renal histopathology as we believe that it is important for clinicians to be able to evaluate such material. We hope also that we have conveyed some of the enthusiasm which we have for this fascinating field of medicine.

Timothy H.J. Goodship
The Royal Victory Infirmary
Newcastle upon Tyne, UK

Bradley J. Maroni
Emery University School of Medicine
The Emery Clinic
Atlanta, Georgia, USA

Acknowledgements

We are very grateful to colleagues who have made available many of the illustrations used herein. In particular we thank Sheldon I. Bastacky, A. Capone, Arthur Greenberg, R. Hennigar, K. Hewan-Lowe, Brenda Lee Holbert, Adrian Morley, Raymond M. Rault, V. Silva and A. Someren. We also thank Drs Pai and Heywood, the *New England Journal of Medicine* and Peritoneal Dialysis International for allowing us to reproduce material that has already been published.

Contributors

John Brock III, MD
Associate Professor of Surgery and
Director of Pediatric Urology
Vanderbilt University Medical
Center, Nashville, Tennessee, USA

Alison Brown, MD, MRCP
Consultant Nephrologist
Freeman Hospital, Newcastle upon
Tyne, UK

Brian England, MD
Associate Professor of Medicine
Renal Division, Emory University
School of Medicine, Atlanta,
Georgia, USA

John Feehally, MA, DM, FRCP
Consultant Nephrologist
Leicester General Hospital,
Leicester, UK

Antonio Guasch, MD
Assistant Professor of Medicine
Renal Division, Emory University
School of Medicine, Atlanta,
Georgia, USA

James Johnston, MD
Associate Professor of Medicine
Renal Electrolyte Division,
Presbyterian University Hospital,
Pittsburgh, Pennsylvania, USA

Bruce Kaplan, MD
Assistant Professor of Medicine
Division of Nephrology and
Hypertension, Northwestern
University Medical School, Chicago,
Illinois, USA

Bertram Kasiske, MD
Professor of Medicine
Division of Nephrology, Hennepin
County Medical Center,
Minneapolis, Minnesota, USA

Carl Kjellstrand, MD, PhD
Professor of Medicine
University of Alberta, Edmonton,
Alberta, Canada

Brian Ling, MD
Associate Professor of Medicine
Renal Division, Emory University
School of Medicine, Atlanta,
Georgia, USA

John Neylan, MD
Associate Professor of Medicine,and
Medical Director, Renal
Transplantation
Emory University School of
Medicine, Atlanta, Georgia, USA

Stuart Rodger, MB, FRCP
Consultant Nephrologist,
Western Infirmary, Glasgow, UK

Contributors

Kim Solez, MD
Professor of Pathology and Director
of Lab Medicine and Pathology
University of Alberta, Edmonton,
Alberta, Canada

John Tapson, BSc, MD, FRCP
Consultant Nephrologist
Freeman Hospital, Newcastle upon
Tyne, UK

Paul Warwicker, BSc, MRCP
Research Fellow
University of Newcastle upon Tyne,
Newcastle upon Tyne, UK

Robert Wilkinson, BSc, MD, FRCP
Professor of Renal Medicine and
Consultant Nephrologist
Freeman Hospital, Newcastle upon
Tyne, UK

1 A 24-year-old cadaveric renal transplant recipient was doing well on maintenance cyclosporin, prednisone, and azathioprine until two months after transplantation. At that time, she was noted to have an acute rise in serum creatinine. A percutaneous allograft biopsy was obtained (**1**).
i. Was it appropriate to obtain a biopsy in this patient?
ii. What does the biopsy show?
iii. How should this patient be treated?

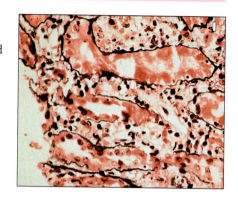

2 This graph (**2**) shows changes in serum creatinine (μmol/l) with time in a patient with chronic pyelonephritis.
i. What is the scale of the serum creatinine?
ii. Why is there a progressive decline in renal function?

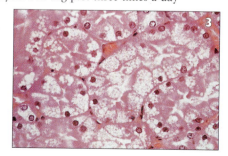

3 You are asked to evaluate a 35-year-old man who three years previously had received a cadaveric renal transplant for chronic renal failure secondary to IgA nephropathy; post-operatively the baseline creatinine stabilised at 1.9 mg/dl (170 μmol/l) on cyclosporin, azathioprine and prednisone. One week prior to admission the patient developed low-grade fever and a productive cough. He was seen by his family physician and erythromycin 333 mg p.o. three times a day prescribed. His symptoms resolved, but on the day prior to admission he noted a decrease in urine output. His serum creatinine was 6.0 mg/dl (530 μmol/l), trough cyclosporin level was 250 ng/ml (whole blood HPLC), and a renal transplant biopsy obtained (**3**).
i. What does the renal biopsy show?
ii. What is the cause of this problem?
iii. What is the appropriate therapy?

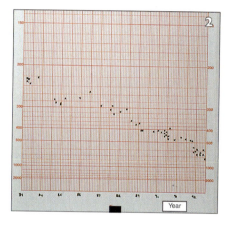

1 i. The differential diagnosis of an acute rise in serum creatinine includes acute rejection, cyclosporin (CSA) nephrotoxicity, ureteral obstruction and other less common disorders. Although patients can sometimes be treated empirically, there are advantages to obtaining an allograft biopsy as soon as a rise in serum creatinine is confirmed. This approach avoids potentially harmful delays in therapy and allows treatment to be tailored to the severity of the biopsy findings. In addition, a biopsy can help to diagnose acute CSA toxicity, thereby avoiding unnecessary immunosuppression.
ii. This biopsy shows invasion of the renal tubular epithelium with mononuclear cells, or so-called tubulitis. It is indicative of an acute cellular rejection.
iii. Most episodes of acute cellular rejection respond to a course of high-dose corticosteroids. Sometimes, more potent immunosuppressive agents, such as the monoclonal antibody OKT3, are necessary.

2 i. The serum creatinine has been plotted on a reciprocal scale because serum creatinine has an inverse relationship with glomerular filtration rate (GFR).
ii. The reason for the progressive decline in renal function in patients with established chronic renal failure is probably multifactorial, including ongoing activity of the primary renal disease, hypertension, hyperlipidaemia and hyperfiltration in the remnant nephrons. Optimal control of blood pressure and restriction of dietary protein may delay the rate of progression. Angiotensin-converting enzyme inhibitors (ACEIs) are the antihypertensive agents of choice , as they have an additional benefit in slowing the rate of progression.

3 i. The renal biopsy demonstrates isometric vacuolisation of the renal tubules caused by acute cyclosporin nephrotoxicity. This type of damage is usually subacute and is associated with vacuolisation, proximal tubule microcalcification, tubular atrophy and accumulation of giant mitochondria in the tubules. Similar changes can also be seen with acute tacrolimus (FK 506) nephrotoxicity.
ii. Acute nephrotoxicity in this patient resulted from the increase in cyclosporin levels caused by the competitive inhibition of cyclosporin metabolism by the hepatic cytochrome P450 system produced by erythromycin. It is well-established that erythromycin, diltiazem, verapamil, nicardipine, metoclopramide, corticosteroids and ketoconazole increase cyclosporin levels. Conversely, drugs such as isoniazid, rifampicin, phenytoin and phenobarbital induce hepatic enzymes, accelerating cyclosporin metabolism and decreasing its blood levels. Failure to recognise these drug interactions can increase the risk of rejection or cyclosporin nephrotoxicity.

Finally, nephrotoxins such as aminoglycosides, melphalan, amphotericin B and ketoconazole may increase the risk of nephrotoxicity when administered concomitantly with cyclosporin.
iii. Stop the erythromycin and monitor cyclosporin blood levels. In patients on immunosuppressive drugs it is particularly important to recognise potential drug interactions and to closely monitor blood levels when drugs with known interactions are administered.

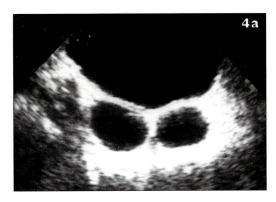

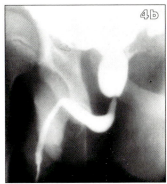

4 A 4-year-old boy is referred because of a weak urine stream and failure to thrive. The child is in the fifth percentile for height and on physical examination a suprapubic mass is palpable. What investigations have been undertaken (**4a, 4b**) and what do they show?

5 A 45-year old man complained of nausea, vomiting, haematuria and severe right flank pain radiating to his groin. He denied having fever, dysuria, urethral discharge, urgency, hesitancy or incontinence. The patient had chronic diarrhoea from irritable bowel syndrome, but no history of gout. His blood pressure was 140/90 mmHg, heart rate 110 b.p.m., temperature 37.3°C and weight 105 kg. He had right flank tenderness, but the remainder of his examination was unremarkable. An IVP revealed a radiolucent filling defect in his right ureter. The patient received analgesics and intravenous fluids, and spontaneously passed a renal calculus which was sent for analysis. The results of two 24-hour urine collections obtained while consuming his usual diet are shown (Table).
i. What are the possible causes of his nephrolithiasis?
ii. Why did this patient develop a kidney stone?
iii. What therapy should be recommended?

Test	Usual diet	Usual diet	Units	Reference values
Volume	940	860	ml	–
pH	5.5	5.5	–	–
Calcium	156	103	mg/day	<250 mg/day (males)
Uric acid	420	330	mg/day	<750 mg/day
Creatinine	1950	1800	mg/day	–
Sodium	284	174	mmol/day	–
Magnesium	8.6	6.0	mEq/day	>5 mEq/day
Oxalate	34	36	mg/day	<40 mg/day
Citrate	130	80	mg/day	>250 mg/day

4 An abdominal ultrasound examination and voiding cystourethrogram (VCUG) have been undertaken. The former confirmed the presence of a markedly enlarged bladder with dilated ureters visible posterior to the bladder (**4a**) and the latter revealed a dilated posterior urethra and enlarged trabeculated bladder (**4b**), a typical finding for a child with posterior urethral valves. His physical examination revealed a distended bladder extending above the umbilicus. Visualisation of the upper urinary tract also revealed bilateral hydronephrosis.

In this setting a VCUG is the diagnostic study of choice. Bladder outlet obstruction is relieved by transurethral incision of the urethral valves. Residual renal function is evaluated by measuring creatinine clearance, and using ultrasonography to assess the residual renal cortex.

5 i. This patient most likely has uric acid nephrolithiasis. Calcium, struvite and cystine stones are radiopaque, whereas uric acid stones are radiolucent. Thus, the radiolucent defect on IVP suggests uric acid nephrolithiasis, which was confirmed by stone analysis. Uric acid is responsible for 5–10% of kidney stones in the US and Northern Europe. It precipitates when the solubility of uric acid decreases and/or when uric acid excretion increases. Uric acid solubility is pH-dependent, with precipitation occurring at a low urine pH. Increased urinary uric acid occurs due to overproduction, increased renal urate excretion or excessive ingestion of dietary purines (diets rich in animal protein).

ii. In spite of a normal urinary uric acid excretion, this man formed uric acid stones because he had a concentrated and acidic urine, precipitated by gastrointestinal fluid and alkali loss from chronic diarrhoea.

iii. A patient with more than one episode of nephrolithiasis should undergo a complete metabolic evaluation, including at least two 24-hour urine collections obtained while the patient consumes his or her usual diet. The urine volume, sodium, uric acid, creatinine, urea, calcium, magnesium, oxalate, citrate and phosphate concentrations should be measured. Treatment for uric acid stones includes:

(a) ensuring a urine volume ≥2 l/day;

(b) reducing dietary purine intake;

(c) increasing uric acid solubility by making the urine more alkaline.

The last can be achieved with either oral sodium bicarbonate or citrate (sodium or potassium salts) and the goal is to maintain the urine pH >6. Sodium bicarbonate is advantageous because it is less expensive, but the additional sodium intake may increase urinary calcium excretion and the risk of calcium stones. Therefore, potassium citrate may be preferable. Allopurinol should be prescribed if these measures fail or if uric acid excretion remains very high (>1000 mg/day).

6 A patient with severe nephrotic syndrome is seen in his physician's office. He has mild hypertension, serum creatinine is 1.8 mg/dl (160 μmol/l), serum albumin is 1.8 g/dl and the 24-hour urine protein is 28 g. Physical examination is notable for 4+ oedema and hepatomegaly. He takes frusemide (furosemide) 80 mg per day, but has recently noted an increase in his weight and worsening oedema. Mechanisms for frusemide resistance in this patient include which of the following:
i. Hypoalbuminaemia.
ii. Albuminuria.
iii. Low effective blood volume.
iv. Increase in distal nephron capacity for Na^+ reabsorption.
v. All of the above.

7 A 1-year-old boy is found to have a urinary tract infection. A renal ultrasound reveals bilateral hydronephrosis, so a VCUG is undertaken.
i. What does the VCUG (**7a**, **7b**) show?
ii. What would be the next step?

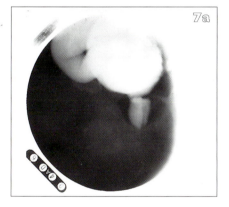
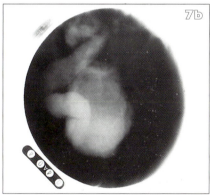

8 This patient, who started CAPD a few days earlier, now complains of inflow pain and poor drainage.
i. What does the radiograph (**8**) show?
ii. What are the possible treatments?

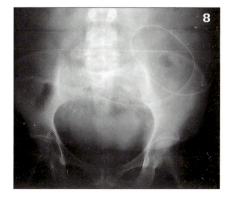

11

6 v. Loop diuretics, including frusemide (furosemide), act by inhibiting the Na–K–2Cl cotransporter in the thick ascending limb of Henle (TALH). For frusemide to have maximal effect, sufficient Na^+ and free frusemide must be delivered to the TALH. If effective blood volume is decreased, such as with severe nephrosis, the proximal reabsorption of sodium and water may increase markedly, thus diminishing distal sodium delivery. Furthermore, the secondary hyperaldosteronic state induced by nephrosis will increase sodium reabsorption by the distal convoluted tubule and cortical collecting duct, further impairing sodium excretion. Frusemide is highly bound to albumin. Since *free* frusemide is necessary to inhibit the Na–K–2Cl cotransporter, freely filtered albumin may 'bind' frusemide within the tubule, rendering it less available to interact with the Na–K–2Cl cotransporter. The high protein binding of frusemide means its volume of distribution is relatively small. As serum albumin falls, less frusemide is protein bound and the volume of distribution increases, decreasing the concentration *delivered* to the nephron. Finally, studies indicate that both distal convoluted tubule and cortical collecting duct Na^+ reabsorption are augmented following chronic frusemide use. Therapeutic strategies which have been used in this setting include administering frusemide with albumin (to decrease the volume of distribution and keep the drug in the intravascular space) and addition of a more distally acting diuretic, e.g. metolazone or spironolactone.

7 i. The VCUG shows a dilated posterior urethra (**7a**), enlarged bladder and massive right-sided ureteral reflux (**7a, 7b**), characteristic of posterior urethral valves. A nuclear renogram shows no renal function on the side with reflux. This has been termed the VURD syndrome (i.e., valves, unilateral reflux and dysplasia). Usually, the contralateral kidney is relatively spared because the bladder is decompressed by the unilateral reflux.
ii. In this child, the urethral valves were incised; if urinary tract infections persist, the affected kidney and ureter may need to be removed.

8 i. This plain abdominal radiograph shows that the curled tip of the continuous ambulatory peritoneal dialysis (CAPD) catheter has migrated out of the pelvis to the left lumbar region. There is also widespread metastatic calcification, including an abdominal aortic aneurysm.
ii. Malposition of the CAPD catheter on the left side may correct itself spontaneously or after a laxative (aperient), if the patient is constipated. If the catheter remains out of position, abdominal discomfort and poor drainage are likely to continue. The catheter tip may move back into the pelvis if the peritoneal cavity is filled with a further 2–4 l of fluid and the patient placed in a head-down position. If this fails, manipulation using a stiff guidewire, laparoscopy or surgery will be required.

9 A 65-year-old man, post abdominal aneurysm repair, is intubated in the intensive care unit. He is receiving nothing p.o. and is on intravenous D_5NS (dextrose/saline) at 50 ml/h. His blood pressure is 100/70 mmHg with pulmonary wedge pressure 12 mmHg and central venous pressure (CVP) 3–5 mmHg. The patient is receiving frusemide (furosemide) 40 mg b.i.d. Laboratory data are given (Table). On day 4, the urine osmolarity was 400 mOsm/l, urine Na^+ 70 mmol/l and urine output is 3 litres.

i. The patient's hypernatraemia is likely due to:
(a) Nephrogenic diabetes.
(b) Unrecorded hypertonic replacement solutions.
(c) Free water deficit induced by frusemide (furosemide) diuresis and normal saline fluid replacement.

ii. What is the free water deficit?
iii. What intravenous fluid regimen would you recommend?

Post-oper-ative day	Serum Na^+ (mmol/l)	BUN		Creatinine		Weight (kg)
		(mg/dl)	(mmol/l)	(mg/dl)	(μmol/l)	
1	140	16	5.7	1.0	88	80
2	147	20	7.1	1.0	88	77
3	155	23	8.2	1.1	97	75
4	161	28	10.0	1.4	124	73

10 This 42-year-old black woman developed a slowly enlarging skin lesion and upper extremity oedema 4 years following renal transplantation.
i. What is the skin lesion shown (**10**)?
ii. What is the appropriate therapy?

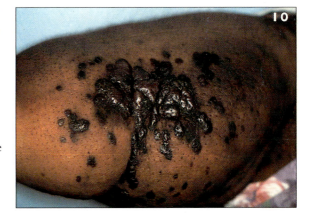

9 i. (c) Patients with free access to water and an intact thirst mechanism will not become hypernatraemic. In this case, the patient was intubated and cannot access water, and so is captive to the intravenous fluids provided by his physicians. This is further aggravated by the impairment of urinary concentrating ability by frusemide (furosemide). The medullary interstitial osmotic gradient favouring water reabsorption is maintained in part by sodium reabsorption in the TALH. Thus, inhibition of the $Na^+–K^+–2Cl^-$ pump in the TALH by frusemide (furosemide) impairs urinary concentrating ability and increases free water losses (hence a urine osmolarity of only 400 mOsm/l). As a rule of thumb, urinary sodium losses with a loop diuretic are typically 60–70 mmol/l or roughly equivalent to 1/2 normal saline (NS). Based on his daily weight loss of 2–3 kg we can estimate that urinary losses are equivalent to 2–3 l. Thus, urinary losses of free H_2O are about 1–1.5 l/day (i.e., 1 litre of 1/2 NS = 0.5 l H_2O and 0.5 l NS). Given his insensible losses, the free water deficit may actually be greater.

ii) The free water deficit can be calculated by [where total body water (TBW) = 0.6 x total body weight]:

(Desired – actual serum [Na^+])/(Desired serum [Na^+]) x TBW = free water deficit

In this patient this is (161 – 140/140) x 80 kg x 0.6 = 7.2 l.

iii) Replacement of one half of the free water deficit during the first 24 hours would be reasonable. This would be in addition to his ongoing losses, e.g., 3 l D_5W and 3 l 1/2 NS, if urine losses remain at their present level.

10 i. The purplish plaques are characteristic of Kaposi's sarcoma. This neoplastic growth, composed of vascular and fibroblastic elements, accounts for approximately 10% of skin malignancies in organ transplant recipients worldwide. In some ethnic groups and regions, such as the eastern Mediterranean area and certain parts of Africa, this lesion is even more common. Putative oncogenic viruses may account for its increased frequency in immunocompromised populations, such as AIDS and transplant patients.

ii. Withdrawal of immunosuppression is usually required, especially if there is visceral involvement. In addition, radiation therapy and chemotherapy may be warranted.

11 i. What is this device (11)?
ii. What current clinical applications does it have?

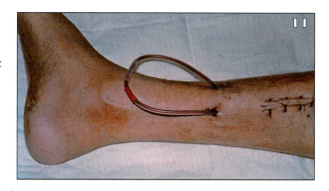

12 This renal biopsy (12) is from a patient with IgA nephropathy who has developed acute renal failure.
i. What is the cause of the acute renal failure?
ii. Why else may a patient with IgA nephropathy develop acute renal failure?

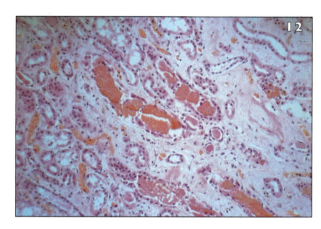

13 This patient developed acute dyspnoea 3 weeks after starting CAPD.
i. What is the most likely cause of the radiological appearances (13) and how should this be confirmed?
ii. What are the treatment options?

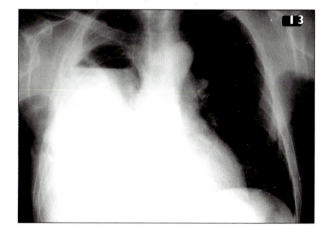

11 i. This is a Scribner shunt.
ii. First described in 1960, the Scribner shunt provided reliable vascular access, permitting the establishment of chonic haemodialysis programmes for the treatment of end-stage renal failure. Although prone to clotting, infection, dislodgement and haemorrhage, the external shunt is still occasionally used as access for continuous arteriovenous haemofiltration (CAVH) or continuous arteriovenous haemodialysis (CAVHD).

12 i. The renal biopsy shows tubular occlusion by blood during an episode of frank haematuria. This is surprisingly uncommon, even in those patients who have recurrent episodes of very heavy haematuria.
ii. The glomerular lesion may undergo transformation into a necrotising crescentic glomerulonephritis – haematuria will not be so heavy and the urine sediment will be active, but this is unusual in IgA nephropathy.

13 i. It is very likely that this patient has developed a communication between the peritoneal and pleural cavities resulting in an acute hydrothorax. This is nearly always right-sided and the diagnosis is confirmed by finding a high glucose concentration in a diagnostic aspirate of the effusion.
ii. Drainage of the peritoneal cavity should ameliorate breathlessness and peritoneal dialysis should be discontinued. A permanent change to haemodialysis should be considered, but if this is not appropriate CAPD should not be restarted until the defect has been repaired or sealed. Contrast or isotope peritonography has been used to locate the site of pleuroperitoneal communication with mixed success.
Intrapleural instillation of tetracycline, talc and autologous blood have been reported in some cases to cause effective pleurodesis. The defect may also be repaired following a mini thoracotomy or by laparoscopic surgery.

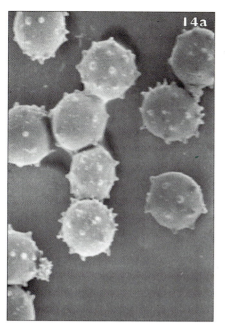

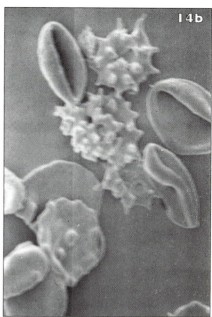

14 Shown (**14a, 14b**) are scanning electron micrographs of erythrocytes present in the urine of two patients with microscopic haematuria. Where is the likely origin of the bleeding in each case?

15 A transplant recipient, who was receiving CSA, prednisone and azathioprine, developed hypertension and proteinuria 18 months after transplantation. Treatment was begun with an ACEI, and several weeks later these laboratory tests (Table) were obtained.
i. Which laboratory abnormalities may have been caused, at least in part, by the ACEI?
ii. Should ACEIs be avoided in renal transplant recipients?

Test	Result
Haemoglobin	10.0 g/dl
Creatinine	2.6 mg/dl (230 μmol/l)
Sodium	141 mmol/l
Potassium	5.9 mmol/l
Chloride	119 mmol/l
Total CO_2	17 mmol/l

14 Assessment of the morphology of urine erythrocytes can be helpful diagnostically. Red blood cells that originate from the glomeruli (glomerular bleeding) are exposed to physical and osmotic trauma during their passage along the nephron. Consequently, the erythrocytes typically vary in size, shape and haemoglobin content (**14b**). Non-glomerular bleeding from sites distal to the ducts of Bellini shows a much more uniform erythrocyte appearance (**14a**). This simple test can quickly guide further investigation of the patient with microscopic haematuria.

Unfortunately, such assessment is often difficult with simple light microscopy (particularly with an inexperienced observer), so phase contrast or scanning electron microscopy is necessary to differentiate between glomerular and non-glomerular bleeding. In experienced hands, phase contrast microscopy is 100% sensitive and 90% specific at diagnosing glomerular bleeding for both children and adults. Alternatively, an automated red cell analyser can be used to measure the cell volumes of the urinary erythrocytes, which correlates well with the underlying pathology, non-glomerular bleeding tending to be associated with the presence of larger red cells in the urine. This method predicts a non-glomerular source of the haematuria with a sensitivity of 81% and a specificity of 100%.

Although glomerulonephritis is usually associated with polymorphic and distorted erythrocytes in the urine, occasionally a mixed population of cells may be seen. In the acute phase of post-streptococcal glomerulonephritis, for example, some 80–90% of the erythrocytes may be of uniform appearance.

15 i. ACEIs can lower haemoglobin levels in renal transplant recipients and may have contributed to this patient's mild anaemia. ACEIs can also cause an increase in serum creatinine, especially in patients with renal artery stenosis or intrarenal vascular disease seen in chronic rejection, presumably by lowering intraglomerular pressure. Hyperkalaemia is a common complication of ACEI therapy, especially in renal transplant patients in whom mild type IV renal tubular acidosis is common. Often the hyperkalaemia can be treated by adding a loop diuretic, the addition of which can potentiate the antihypertensive effects of the ACEI as well.
ii. Serious adverse effects of ACEIs are unusual, and there are both practical and theoretical advantages to ACEI therapy in renal transplant recipients. Therefore, ACEIs may be used in renal transplant recipients, as long as these individuals are closely monitored for potential adverse effects.

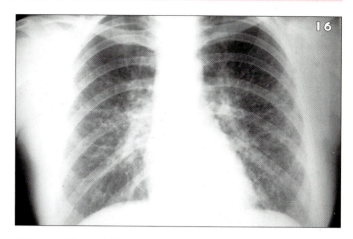

16 A middle-aged black man presented with fever, weight loss, progressive dyspnoea and a non-productive cough. On examination, he had tender red nodules on the anterior surface of his legs, dry eyes and diffuse lung crackles. Serum chemistries are unremarkable, except for a serum creatinine of 1.8 mg/dl (160 µmol/l). The chest radiograph is shown (16) and KUB revealed nephrocalcinosis. What is the most likely diagnosis?

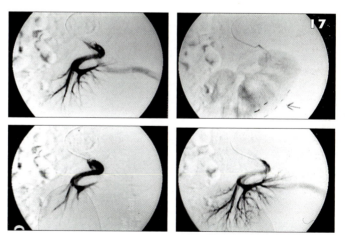

17 Five years after a mismatched cadaveric renal transplant, a patient developed a gradual rise in serum creatinine, nephrotic range proteinuria and worsening hypertension. An ACEI was added to the regimen and shortly thereafter his renal function declined further. What is demonstrated on this arteriogram (17)?

16 The chest radiograph shows a miliary lung infiltrate, which may be present in a variety of diseases (i.e., lymphoma, tuberculosis or fungal infections). The combination of skin, eye and lung involvement, as well as nephrocalcinosis, suggests the possibility of sarcoidosis.

Sarcoidosis is a systemic disease attributed to an exaggerated cellular immune response to an unknown antigen(s). Hyperactive helper T cells release inflammatory mediators that participate in the recruitment and activation of blood monocytes, resulting in granuloma formation and organ dysfunction. Sarcoidosis usually presents in young and middle-aged individuals. The lung is the organ most commonly involved (90% of cases), typically with a reticulonodular pattern visible on chest radiographs. Lymphadenopathy of the pulmonary hilum and paratracheal regions is very common. Skin involvement occurs in the form of erythema nodosum, skin plaques, maculopapular rashes and subcutaneous nodules. Uveitis is seen in 25% of patients with sarcoidosis. Lacrimal gland involvement with a keratoconjunctivitis sicca can also occur. Histological evidence of liver damage is present in two-thirds of patients, but it is usually not clinically important. The most common renal abnormalities are hypercalciuria, which may result in hypercalcaemia, tubular functional abnormalities and nephrocalcinosis. In biopsy and autopsy series the prevalence of renal involvement varies from 15–40%. A granulomatous interstitial nephritis is typically seen; the glomeruli are usually normal or show only mild mesangial widening. Immunofluorescence is negative.

17 The arteriogram demonstrates the obliterative vasculopathy characteristic of chronic rejection. There is a dramatic pruning of the renal vasculature, especially in the cortex associated with microaneurysms. While an ACEI may be beneficial in reducing proteinuria, care should be taken in its administration. The attendant reduction in intraglomerular pressures may lead to an acute reduction in GFR, similar to that seen with renal artery stenosis. In this instance, the ACEI was discontinued and the serum creatinine returned to baseline.

18 A 35-year-old woman who is known to have a mitral valve prolapse is admitted with general malaise and a fever. Three blood cultures yield a significant growth of *Staphylococcus aureus*. Treatment is started with intravenous fluloxacillin and ceftazidime. Over the next week, the serum urea increases from 22 to 56 mg/dl (8 to 20 mmol/l) and the creatinine from 1.6 to 4.0 mg/dl

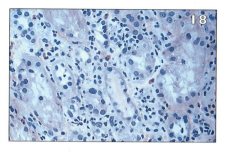

(140 to 350 μmol/l). Urinalysis on day 7 reveals proteinuria ++ and blood ++, urine microscopy shows red blood cells, white blood cells, granular casts and white cell casts. A renal biopsy is undertaken (**18**).
i. What is the differential diagnosis?
ii. What does the renal biopsy show?
iii. What other investigations would be useful in establishing the diagnosis?

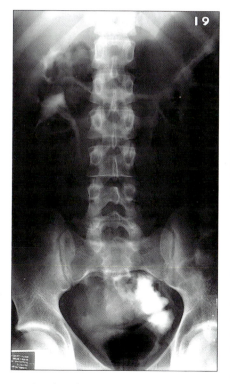

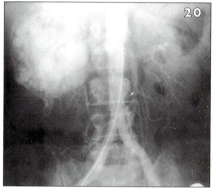

20 A young man was noted to have an epididymal swelling during his army service which was removed surgically. He subsequently developed macroscopic haematuria which was investigated by angiography (**20**). His blood pressure was 194/112 mmHg and fundoscopy showed AV nipping and an angioma.
i. What does the angiogram show?
ii. What was the likely nature of the epididymal swelling?
iii. What are the other features of this syndrome and how should they be investigated?

19 i. What does this IVP (**19**) show?
ii. What are the complications of this?

18 i. The differential diagnosis of acute renal failure in this patient includes post-infectious acute glomerulonephritis, drug-induced interstitial nephritis and ischaemic tubular necrosis.
ii. The biopsy shows a dense interstitial infiltrate of neutrophils, lymphocytes and eosinophils diagnostic of interstitial nephritis. An interstitial infiltrate can be seen with acute tubular necrosis, but it is less pronounced and eosinophils are not seen. Allergic interstitial nephritis (AIN) usually follows 7–10 days of drug treatment and may be seen with many medications, including penicillins, cephalosporins, sulphonamides, rifampicin and thiazide diuretics
iii. Investigations that might have assisted in the diagnosis include a differential white cell count (showing eosinophilia), serum complement levels (decreased in post-infectious glomerulonephritis) and urine cytology (looking for eosinophils which may be seen in interstitial nephritis). The mainstay of treatment is withdrawal of the offending agent. The use of corticosteroids is controversial; they may hasten recovery of renal function, but they do not appear to improve long-term outcome.

19 i. This IVP shows a ureterosigmoidostomy which is a urinary diversion procedure that has largely been superseded by the ileal conduit.
ii. The complications of a uterosigmoidostomy include hyperchloraemic metabolic acidosis with hypokalaemia, osteomalacia, diarrhoea due to incontinence of urine from the rectum, reflux of faecal material causing infection, interstitial nephritis and scarring. A late complication is the development of adenomas and carcinomas at the site of the ureteric anastamosis. The cells of the colon are capable of reabsorption of water and electrolytes; in this case chloride ions are exchanged for bicarbonate which results in a normal anion gap acidosis. Increased fluid delivery stimulates potassium secretion by the sigmoid colon, causing hypokalaemia.

20 i. The angiogram shows a large vascular tumour replacing the right kidney. The appearances are consistent with a hypernephroma.
ii. The epididymal swelling is likely to be a cystadenoma.
iii. The features of this case are consistent with a diagnosis of Von Hippel–Lindau syndrome. Other features include retinal angiomatosis, cerebellar haemangioblastomas, spinal cord angiomas, phaeochromocytoma and pancreatic tumours. The following should therefore be included in the regular follow-up of these patients; fundoscopy, CT or MRI of the head, renal ultrasound and measurement of urinary catecholamines.

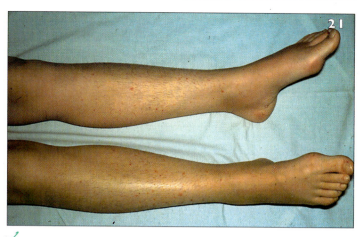

21 This adolescent patient had recurrent crops of spots on the legs (mainly extensor surfaces, **21**) and arms. The patient also had arthralgias, episodic abdominal pain and microscopic haematuria.
i. What is the probable diagnosis?
ii. How would you confirm the diagnosis?
iii. Could the renal biopsy appearance in IgA nephropathy (see **49**) be consistent with this diagnosis?

22 A 43-year-old man has had one or two episodes of renal colic annually for the past 4 years. One of the stones was composed of calcium oxalate, so he was told to follow a low-calcium diet. His father, brother and two uncles have had kidney stones. The patient takes no medications and his physical examination was normal. Serum chemistries were normal and two 24-hour urines collected while eating his usual diet are given (Table).

Test	Usual diet	Usual diet	Units	Reference values
Volume	1580	1240	ml	–
pH	4.5	6.5	–	–
Calcium	340	400	mg/day	<250 mg/day (males)
Phosphorus	960	1240	mg/day	–
Uric acid	243	630	mg/day	<750 mg/day
Creatinine	1800	1800	mg/day	–
Urea nitrogen	12.9	14.5	g/day	–
Sodium	100	120	mmol/day	–
Magnesium	7.7	10.0	mEq/day	>5 mEq/day
Oxalate	41	38	mg/day	<40 mg/day
Citrate	1260	1360	mg/day	>250 mg/day

i. What metabolic abnormalities contribute to his nephrolithiasis?
ii. What therapy would you prescribe?

21 i. <u>Henoch–Schönlein purpura</u> (HSP), a term that is a misnomer which persists in clinical use. The rash is vasculitic rather than purpuric, as HSP is a type of small vessel vasculitis.
ii. The diagnosis is confirmed by identifying tissue deposition of IgA (e.g., in skin or renal biopsy). In paediatric practice the diagnosis is often made clinically; this is an appropriate approach, since other forms of systemic vasculitis are very uncommon in children and most episodes of HSP are self-limiting and do not require immunosuppressive treatment.
iii. Yes, the light microscopic appearance is the same in IgA nephropathy and HSP. Focal segmental necrotising glomerulonephritis with crescent formation is less common in IgA nephropathy than in HSP, but is also much less common in HSP than in other forms of small vessel vasculitis which form the differential diagnosis (e.g., Wegener's granulomatosis and microscopic polyarteritis). There is no known explanation for this.
Many now regard IgA nephropathy and HSP as two ends of one spectrum, i.e., IgA nephropathy is a *forme fruste* of HSP – 'HSP without the rash'.

22 i. This man has hypercalciuria, low urine volumes, high protein intake and borderline oxalate excretion. Hypercalciuria is the most common metabolic abnormality to cause nephrolithiasis. The factors responsible for hypercalciuria are enhanced gastrointestinal absorption, increased renal excretion, bone resorption and high dietary sodium intake. High-protein diets are typically purine-rich and therefore increase uric acid excretion, which can act as a nidus for calcium stone formation. Additionally, a high-protein diet lowers urinary pH and urinary citrate excretion. The low urine volume increases the concentration of calcium and oxalate, favouring stone formation.
ii. His diet should be modified to reduce protein, sodium and oxalate intake. Oxalate-rich foods should be limited: e.g., rhubarb, spinach, peanuts, okra, chocolate and tea. In conjunction with a low-sodium diet, a thiazide diuretic will reduce his calcium excretion and hypercalciuria. A low-calcium diet should generally be *avoided* since it may increase oxalate excretion and actually promote stone formation. In addition, low-calcium diets may lead to negative calcium balance in patients with hypercalciuria and increase the risk of osteoporosis.

23 This 59-year-old renal transplant recipient developed unilateral periocular vesicular lesions and conjunctivitis associated with blurred vision and pain. He had enjoyed 5 years of stable graft function and had felt well until the present illness. What is the lesion shown in **23**?

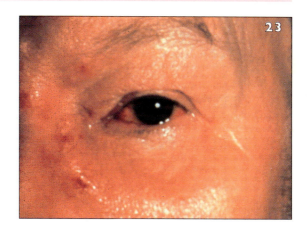

24 A middle-aged woman is admitted because of polyuria, hypotension and moderate renal insufficiency. On admission, the fractional excretion of Na was 3%. She required large volumes of crystalloid and a high salt diet to maintain her blood pressure. Because of renal insufficiency, a kidney biopsy was performed (**24**, courtesy of K. Hewan-Lowe, MD). What is the diagnosis?

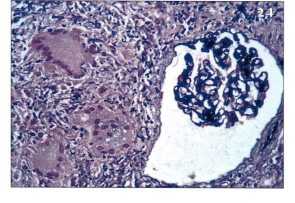

25 A patient had normal renal function and was doing well until 5 weeks after transplantation when her temperature rose to 41°C and the laboratory tests shown (Table) were obtained. What disease would most likely explain these laboratory abnormalities?

Test	Result
WBC	2.1×10^9/l
Haemoglobin	8.8 g/dl
Serum creatinine	2.0 mg/dl (177 µmol/l)
AST	82 U/l
ALT	132 U/l

23 *Herpes zoster* infection may occur any time following transplantation, although reactivation of this latent virus is more likely during periods of increased immuno-suppression. Dermatomal involvement is typical and dissemination is rare. When it involves the ophthalmic branch of the trigeminal nerve, morbidity is considerable and corneal scarring may result. Aggressive therapy is warranted in these cases, utilising both topical and systemic acyclovir.

24 The kidney biopsy (**24**) shows several interstitial non-caseating granulomas, surrounded by lymphocytes and macrophages, with an associated interstitial inflammatory infiltrate and fibrosis, suggestive of sarcoidosis. Nephrocalcinosis secondary to hypercalcaemia or interstitial nephritis are the most common renal lesions seen in sarcoidosis. Estimates for the prevalence of interstitial involvement in sarcoidosis range from 10–40%. The clinical presentation is one of progressive renal insufficiency and tubular dysfunction. Sodium or potassium wasting, glycosuria, nephrogenic diabetes insipidus and proximal or distal renal tubular acidosis may be seen. Kidney size is typically normal, although they may be enlarged. Gallium scans show increased renal uptake, but lack specificity. Serum ACE levels are usually increased in sarcoidosis, but have a low sensitivity and are not very useful for monitoring the efficacy of treatment. Glomerular involvement in sarcoidosis is rare. Membranous, membranoproliferative and focal segmental glomerulosclerosis have been described. The treatment of choice is corticosteroids, which are effective in normalising hypercalcaemia and improving GFR.

25 For each of these laboratory findings there is a long list of differential diagnoses. However, the occurrence of all of the above laboratory findings in the same patient should suggest CMV, especially if it occurs shortly after transplantation. CMV infection is typically associated with neutropenia, and often causes mild hepatocellular damage. Anaemia may also be seen, especially if gastrointestinal bleeding occurs. The elevated creatinine, if acute, could be due to dehydration. However, allograft rejection (often associated with CMV infection), CSA nephrotoxicity or (rarely) direct renal involvement from CMV should be considered.

26 i. This patient is on CAPD. What is shown in **26**?
ii. What associated abnormalities may be present?

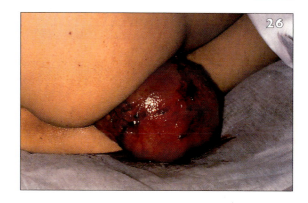

27 A couple's first infant died at 1 year of age from complications of 'kidney and liver disease'. The couple were told that each of their offspring would have a 25% chance of having the same disease and a 50% chance of being a carrier. At the newly expectant parents' request, ultrasonography was performed at 35 weeks' gestation. The ultrasound (**27**) reveals the foetus to have markedly enlarged echogenic kidneys (k), oligohydramnios (H) and

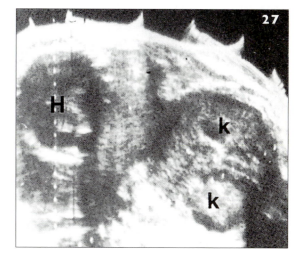

an empty urinary bladder. The father (32 years old) and mother (31 years old) have been in excellent health. Which of the following should the paediatric nephrologist suspect?
i. Medullary cystic disease.
ii. Autosomal dominant polycystic kidney disease (ADPKD).
iii. Tuberous sclerosis.
iv. Autosomal recessive polycystic kidney disease (ARPKD).
v. Von Hippel–Lindau syndrome.

26 i. This CAPD patient has a prolapsed rectum, an unusual complication of peritoneal dialysis precipitated by raised intra-abdominal pressure and loss of tone in the pelvic floor muscles.

ii. Over 10% of patients develop abdominal hernias after starting treatment with CAPD. While usually clinically obvious and most often situated at incisional, umbilical and inguinal sites, small strangulated and Richter's hernias may occasionally be missed or mistaken for CAPD peritonitis. Oedema of the abdominal wall and genitalia, respiratory dysfunction and acute hydrothorax are other complications of the raised intra-abdominal pressure which accompanies peritoneal dialysis.

27 iv. ARPKD or infantile polycystic kidney disease, the clinical manifestations of which include varying degrees of renal and hepatic involvement. ARPKD occurs in 1:10,000 to 1:40,000 births and is due to a genetic defect located on chromosome 6. Renal manifestations include impaired diluting and concentrating ability, distal renal tubular acidosis, hypertension and renal failure, usually progressing to end-stage renal disease (ESRD) after 5–15 years. Liver manifestations include hepatic cysts and fibrosis producing portal hypertension, and dilatation of intrahepatic and biliary ducts predisposing to cholangitis.

As here, the diagnosis can be made in severe cases by antenatal ultrasonography after 24 weeks' gestation. Such a presentation is usually accompanied by pulmonary hypoplasia and/or insufficiency and early death. However, infants surviving beyond their first month of life have a >80% probability of living past 15 years of age. In children with less severe expression, ARPKD can be documented by renal ultrasound (or CT scan) which shows progressive enlargement of the kidneys (>2 standard deviations above normal), increased echogenicity and multiple small cysts (<3 mm). Since the phenotypic expression of ARPKD may vary within families, asymptomatic siblings of children with newly diagnosed ARPKD should be evaluated for clinically 'silent' renal and hepatic involvement. Renal histology reveals cortical cysts originating from dilatation of the collecting ducts.

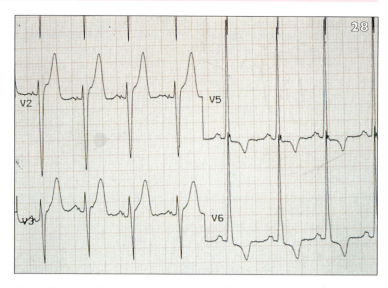

28 A 38-year-old man is found to have a blood pressure of 190/115 mmHg at an insurance medical examination. A repeat measurement of 166/112 mmHg is obtained by his family physician. An ECG is performed (**28**).

i. What does the ECG show?

ii. Describe another method to assess the effects of hypertension on the heart and compare its sensitivity to electrocardiography.

iii. What is the prognostic significance of the ECG changes?

29 A 27-year-old Caucasian woman was well until 35 weeks into her second pregnancy (her first pregnancy had been uncomplicated), when she developed anorexia, nausea and vomiting and became jaundiced. Her blood pressure was 150/95 mmHg and she had no proteinuria. Laboratory investigations were: bilirubin 5.9 mg/dl (102 mmol/l), ALT 144 IU/l, alkaline phosphatase 295 IU/l, albumin 29 g/l, platelets 109 x 10^9/l, prothrombin time 16 s, creatinine 1.8 mg/dl (157 μmol/l). She had an urgent caesarian section, delivering a healthy infant. Two days post-partum her conscious level deteriorated and oliguria was noted. The platelet count decreased to 42 x 10^9/l and the prothrombin time increased to 26 s. Serum amylase was elevated at 1346 IU/l. What diagnoses should be considered?

28 i. The ECG shows increased voltage, ST depression and T wave inversion in the left ventricular leads. The increased voltage is due to hypertrophy of the left ventricle. The ST depression and T wave inversion are due to reversed left ventricular repolarisation.
ii. Echocardiography is a more sensitive method of detecting left ventricular hypertrophy than ECG.
iii. Patients with hypertension and left ventricular hypertrophy have an increased mortality compared to those with hypertension alone. In hypertensive patients, ECG evidence of left ventricular hypertrophy has the same prognostic value as a previous myocardial infarct.

29 The differential diagnosis includes idiopathic acute fatty liver of pregnancy, HELLP syndrome (haemolysis, elevated liver enzymes and low platelets) and pre-eclampsia with hepatic involvement. Acute fatty liver of pregnancy usually begins in the last trimester, most commonly after the 35th week. There is an increased incidence in primigravidae (especially in twin pregnancies). Nausea, vomiting and abdominal pain are rapidly followed by jaundice and hepatic encephalopathy. Peripheral oedema, hypertension and proteinuria are present in 30–50% of cases and renal failure may occur in about 60%. The platelet count is low, prothrombin time raised and fibrinogen concentration decreased; bilirubin and alkaline phosphatase levels are markedly raised, but transaminases are usually only mildly elevated. Acute pancreatitis is a recognised complication. There is a 10% maternal mortality and 20% foetal mortality.

HELLP syndrome is more common in older Caucasian multigravida women. Transaminase levels are usually modestly increased, bilirubin level is characteristically normal and the platelet count is low. HELLP syndrome may occur without hypertension and proteinuria, and is not associated with acute pancreatitis.

Severe pre-eclampsia is often associated with hepatic dysfunction, as evidenced by a rise in transaminases. Bilirubin is usually normal unless there is haemolysis or hepatic infarction. Severe hypertension and proteinuria are common, but acute pancreatitis is not usually associated. This patient most probably had acute fatty liver of pregnancy complicated by acute pancreatitis, though acute pancreatitis complicated by hepatic dysfunction and disseminated intravascular coagulation is also a possibility. It is possible that acute fatty liver of pregnancy, HELLP and pre-eclampsia with associated hepatic dysfunction are all part of the spectrum of the same clinical entity.

30 i. At a pH of 7.40, what is the [H⁺] concentration?
ii. At a pH of 7.40 and a pCO_2 of 20 mmHg, what is the $[HCO_3^-]$ concentration?
iii. With a pCO_2 of 30 mmHg and a HCO_3^- of 20 mEq/l, what is the blood pH?

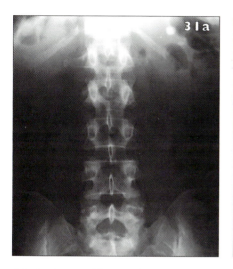
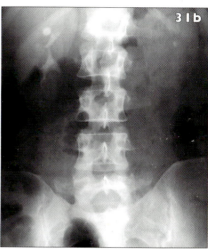

31 A 60-year-old man who was referred with hypertension is found to have a total calcium of 11.4 mg/dl (2.85 mmol/l). He had passed a renal calculus 2 years previously. His plain abdominal radiograph and IVP are shown (**31a, 31b**).
i. What do the radiographs show?
ii. How would you investigate the hypercalcaemia?
iii. What is the relationship between hypercalcaemia and hypertension?

32 This ambulatory blood pressure recording (**32**) is taken from a 26-year-old man who, over a 3-month period, has had several blood pressure measurements over 150/100 mmHg taken by his family physician. What does the recording demonstrate?

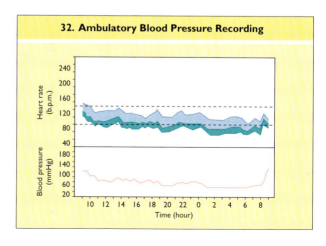

32. Ambulatory Blood Pressure Recording

30 pH is equal to the negative log of [H^+]. The predominant extracellular buffer is HCO_3^-, where $H^+ + HCO_3^- \Leftrightarrow H_2CO_3 \Leftrightarrow H_2O + CO_2$. The relationship of pH to [HCO_3^-] and pCO_2 can be described by the Henderson–Hasselbalch equation:

pH = 6.10 + log ([HCO_3^-]/0.03pCO_2)

To solve for [H^+], the modified equation below can be used.

[H^+] = 24(pCO_2/HCO_3^-)

These equations are useful for evaluating clinical acid–base disturbances and for checking the validity of the blood gas results sent from the clinical laboratory. Potential problems in blood gas collection include loss of pCO_2 if the ABG is not collected anaerobically or failure to keep the blood properly chilled, which may enhance glycolysis and lower pH. Heparin remaining in the syringe may also lower the pH.

i. [H^+] = 40 nmol/l at a pH of 7.40

ii. [HCO_3^-] = 24pCO_2/[H^+] = 24 x 20/40 = 12 mEq/l

iii. [H^+] = 24pCO_2/[HCO_3^-] = 24 x 30/20 = 36 nmol/l

By interpolation, a H^+ concentration of 36 nmol/l is halfway between a pH of 7.4 (H^+ = 40 nmol/l) and pH of 7.5 (H^+ = 32 nmol/l). Therefore, the pH = 7.45.

31 i. The plain abdominal radiograph (**31a**) shows two calculi in the upper pole of the right kidney and one in the mid-zone of the left kidney. The IVP (**31b**) shows the larger of the right-sided calculi within the kidney and absence of function on the left side. This suggests complete obstruction.

ii. In a patient with a raised total calcium, hypercalcaemia should be confirmed by measurement of the ionised calcium concentration. Serum intact parathyroid hormone (iPTH) concentration should be measured. A raised value in the presence of hypercalcaemia confirms the diagnosis of hyperparathyroidism. A value within the normal range does not exclude this diagnosis because hypercalcaemia should suppress the iPTH concentration. Having excluded hyperparathyroidism the possibility of other conditions, such as sarcoidosis and malignancy, should be considered.

iii. Hypercalcaemia is found in 1% of patients who present with hypertension and has an overall prevalence of 0.5% in the general population, so it is likely that hypercalcaemia is causally related to hypertension. The hypertension associated with hyperparathyroidism is secondary to renal impairment induced by nephrocalcinosis. Parathyroidectomy does not usually cure hypertension, but it does prevent further renal damage.

32 The mean 24-hour blood pressure was 118/80 mmHg. The recording shows evidence of 'white-coat' hypertension, with a significant fall in blood pressure within an hour of the monitor being attached. Besides the detection of 'white-coat' hypertension, ambulatory blood pressure monitoring is also useful in the evaluation of drug resistance, the investigation of symptoms suggestive of hypotension and the evaluation of nocturnal blood pressure changes. It is not certain that 'white-coat' hypertension is completely benign and, although treatment may not be indicated, it is wise to advise repeat ambulatory recordings over the long term.

33 This chest radiograph (33) was obtained from a patient with cytomegalovirus (CMV) infection (see **80**).
i. What is the differential diagnosis?
ii. What is the most likely diagnosis given the overall clinical picture?
iii. How should this patient be managed?

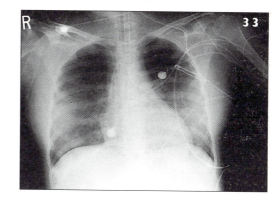

34 A 5-year-old girl is admitted with recurrent urinary infection. Her parents report that she has been incontinent of urine since birth. Shown here (34) is an anatomical abnormality that is responsible for her problem. What is the abnormality?

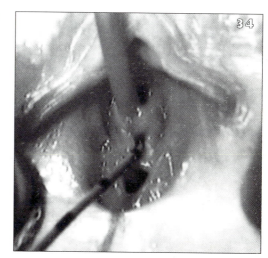

35 This post-mortem specimen (35) shows the kidneys of a man who was treated with haemodialysis for 12 years prior to his death from a cerebrovascular accident. He had developed end-stage renal failure from chronic glomerulonephritis.
i. What abnormality is seen in this pathological specimen?
ii. What complications are associated with this condition?

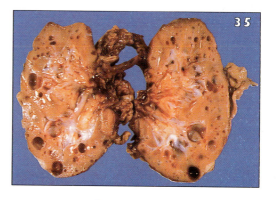

33 i. The list for differential diagnosis of diffuse pulmonary infiltrates in a transplant recipient with fever is long. Viral, bacterial, fungal and protozoan infections could all produce a similar radiograph. Occasionally, lymphoma will present with diffuse pulmonary infiltrates.
ii. Pneumonitis is a common manifestation of CMV, which typically involves multiple organs. CMV pneumonitis can be severe, occasionally leading to respiratory failure and death.
iii. Patients with severe CMV infection are usually treated with a reduction in immunosuppressive medications, intravenous ganciclovir and other supportive measures.

34 In 34 a Foley catheter is located superiorly, an ectopic ureter is cannulated centrally, and the vaginal vestibule is visualised inferiorly. The history is typical for a child with an ectopic ureter, which can drain into numerous locations, most commonly the urethra, vagina, vaginal vestibule or Gartner's duct. Typically, the collecting system is duplicated and the upper pole of the kidney most commonly empties through the ectopic ureter, which is usually severely dysplastic and prone to obstruction and infection. Ultrasonography is the initial study of choice and a duplicated collecting system with hydroureteronephrosis is usually seen. VCUG is performed to ensure that the ectopic ureter does not communicate with the bladder. Finally, cystoscopy and vaginoscopy are performed to evaluate the anatomy and to identify the ectopic ureteral orifice. The renal parenchyma is usually quite dysplastic and, consequently, poor renal function is usually found on a nuclear renogram. Moreover, the contribution of the upper and lower poles of the kidney can also be assessed by nuclear renography. Depending on the degree of residual split renal function (i.e., lower versus upper pole), treatment usually involves either partial nephrectomy of the upper pole or anastomosis of the upper and lower renal pelvis to provide adequate drainage.

35 i. These kidneys demonstrate acquired cystic kidney disease (ACKD). Defined as the development of new cysts in failed kidneys, these changes are seen in both haemodialysis and peritoneal dialysis patients, as well as in patients who are chronically uraemic prior to any dialysis. Incidence, however, increases with time on dialysis, with all patients showing such changes after 8 years of dialysis treatment.
ii. ACKD is usually asymptomatic and not detected without screening or postmortem examination. Flank pain and infection are unusual, but calculus formation is reported. The most frequent complications of ACKD, however, are haemorrhage, erythrocytosis and the development of renal cell carcinoma. Haemorrhage can be significant and occasionally life-threatening. Polycythaemia occurs as a consequence of the production of erythropoietin by the cysts, so the diagnosis should be suspected in any dialysis patient who ceases to require recombinant erythropoietin therapy for anaemia. The most serious risk of ACKD is the development of renal cell carcinoma. Such tumours behave in a similar manner to other renal carcinomas.

36 A transplant recipient developed gradual onset of nocturia and polyuria, associated with a slight rise in serum creatinine.
i. What does the ultrasound (36) show?
ii. What should be done next?

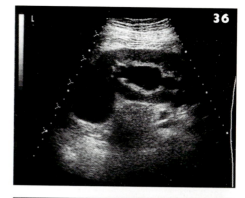

37 A 15-month-old boy is referred with a history of recurrent unexplained fevers and urinary frequency. During the most recent episode urinalysis revealed many white blood cells and urine culture grew a pseudomonas species. On physical examination a left-sided abdominal mass is noted. Following an ultrasound examination, a VCUG is undertaken (37).
i. What do you think the ultrasound examination revealed?
ii. What does the VCUG show?

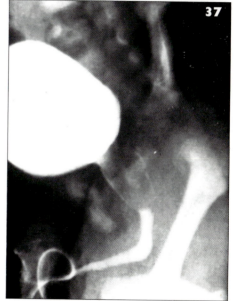

38 This long-term chronic haemodialysis patient developed sudden severe pain in her right heel (38) while walking.
i. What is the diagnosis?
ii. What is the cause of this complication of chronic dialysis?

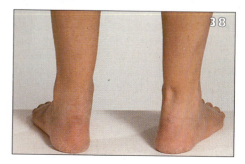

36 i. The renal transplant ultrasound demonstrates moderately severe hydronephrosis. In addition, there is a fluid collection adjacent to the allograft. The character of the echoes within the perinephric fluid collection is consistent with a homogeneous fluid, such as urine or lymph, rather than the complex echoes seen with an abscess or haematoma. The differential diagnosis in this case is urinoma versus lymphocele with ureteral compression. In the former, a urine leak (most often in the distal ureter) results in a localised collection of urine in the abdominal cavity. If there is accompanying outflow obstruction, the progressive resistance causes the collecting system to dilate. In the case of a lymphocele, compression of the ureter may result in hydronephrosis.

ii. A needle aspiration of the fluid collection is the next step. In this case, the finding of proteinaceous fluid containing lymphocytes, rather than an acellular fluid with an elevated creatinine concentration, confirms the presence of lymph rather than urine. Percutaneous drainage resulted in immediate resolution of the hydronephrosis. Lymphoceles may arise from the disrupted lymphatic channels of the donor organ or from the lymphatics of the recipient. Lymphoceles occur in approximately 20% of renal transplant recipients, but usually are asymptomatic. It is only when they compress vital structures that intervention is required. Therapy includes intermittent needle aspiration, prolonged catheter drainage, with or without the use of sclerosing agents, and surgical marsupialisation.

37 i. This history is suggestive of intermittent bladder outlet obstruction, and the abdominal ultrasound reveals a bladder mass which intermittently occludes the urethral orifice. In this case, the mass was fluid-filled and most consistent with a ureterocele. Marked unilateral hydronephrosis was also seen and only a thin rim of renal cortex remained.

ii. VCUG was performed to evaluate the bladder anatomy and to determine whether or not reflux was present. In response to the intermittent obstruction from the ureterocele, ipsilateral ureteral reflux is common, as is present in this case; the contralateral ureter may also reflux secondary to the increased intravesicular pressure. The relative contribution of each kidney to overall renal function is best determined by nuclear renography.

38 i. This patient has developed spontaneous rupture of the Achilles tendon.

ii. Tendon rupture is an unusual problem in dialysis patients; it most frequently involves the quadriceps, triceps or digital tendons. The cause is uncertain, but is believed to be related to weakening of the tendon due to poor blood supply and local calcification. Most patients have biochemical evidence of severe hyperparathyroidism. Advanced uraemia and previous exposure to corticosteroid therapy may also be contributory. Patients may experience discomfort that warns of impending tendon rupture. Rest and treatment of any underlying predisposing factor may be successful in averting rupture. Surgical repair is, however, usually required to treat a broken tendon.

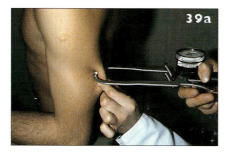

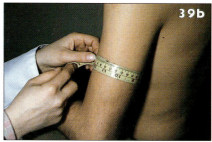

39 **i.** What two measurements (**39a**, **39b**) are being undertaken in this patient with chronic renal failure?
ii. What other parameters can be calculated from these two measurements?
iii. What is the use of these measurements in patients with chronic renal failure?

40 A 5-year-old girl presented with flank pain and hypertension. Work-up revealed microscopic haematuria and mild renal insufficiency. An abdominal ultrasound reveals cysts involving her liver, pancreas and both kidneys. The father (27 years old) and mother (25 years old) are in excellent health and themselves show no evidence of renal cysts on ultrasound. The family history is significant as the paternal grandmother has been on haemodialysis since she 52 years of age. Which of the following should the paediatric nephrologist suspect?
i. Medullary cystic disease.
ii. Tuberous sclerosis.
iii. ARPKD.
iv. Von Hippel–Lindau syndrome.
v. ADPKD.

41 Shown (**41**) is an immuno-
fluorescent stain of a renal
biopsy from a patient who had
recurrent episodes of macroscopic haematuria associated
with upper respiratory tract
infection.
i. What is the diagnosis?
ii. How can an episode of
macroscopic haematuria with
sore throat in this condition be
distinguished clinically from an
episode of post-streptococcal
glomerulonephritis (GN)?

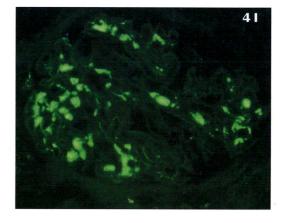

39 i. The triceps skinfold (**39a**) and mid-arm circumference (MAC) (**39b**) are being measured.
ii. From these, arm muscle circumference (AMC) and arm muscle area (AMA) can be calculated. AMC and AMA are indicators of nutritional status, in particular somatic protein stores.
iii. Malnutrition is now established as one of the most important risk factors for mortality in patients with chronic renal failure and it is important that all patients undergo routine nutritional assessment at regular intervals. Other methods commonly used to assess nutritional status include the measurement of dietary intake from 3-day dietary records and urea kinetic modelling (UKM), the measurement of serum albumin and transferrin, and subjective global assessment (SGA).

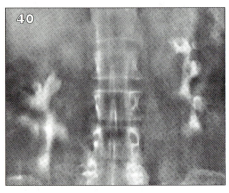

40 v. In contrast to ARPKD, children with ADPKD are usually asymptomatic, with clinical manifestations developing during adulthood. However, affected children may develop microscopic haematuria, hypertension, intracystic infections and renal insufficiency. In children who present with symptoms of ADPKD during the first year of life (50% mortality) and survive, ESRD will develop in about 30%. In less severely affected children, reductions in glomerular filtration rate are usually gradual, with overt renal insufficiency developing after 30 years of age.

Antenatal ultrasonography performed between 30 and 35 weeks of gestation may show hyperechogenic, enlarged kidneys and, occasionally, cysts. In most individuals, bilateral renal cysts will eventually be documented by ultrasound, but may not be apparent before 25–30 years of age. Therefore, younger parents of children with ADPKD may not have detectable renal cysts (in which case grandparents should be screened). In ADPKD, cysts develop in all nephron segments. Intravenous pyelograms show (**40**) multiple radiolucent areas due to renal cysts ('swiss cheese' appearance). Extrarenal cysts (e.g., liver, pancreas, spleen) and cerebral aneurysms have also been described in children with ADPKD.

Finally, ADPKD occurs in 1:400 to 1:1000 births and is due to genetic defects located on chromosome 16 (PKD1), and less commonly chromosome 4.

41 i. IgA nephropathy.
ii. *Timing* – in IgA nephropathy visible haematuria occurs, within 24 hours of the provoking symptoms, whereas in post-infectious GN a delay of 1–3 weeks is typical. *Another distinguishing clinical feature* is that an acute nephritic syndrome typically occurs in post-streptococcal GN, but is very unusual in IgA nephropathy.

42 A 44-year-old dialysis patient received a cadaveric renal allograft within 24 hours of his last dialysis. Admission potassium was 4.7 mmol/l and he tolerated the surgery without difficulty. Initial graft function was poor, with urine output of 60 ml/h. In the recovery room the patient was noted to be hypertensive, so labetolol 15 mg i.v. was administered several times. Several hours later the potassium was 7.0 mmol/l. Serum glucose and arterial blood gas were normal. An electro-cardiogram was

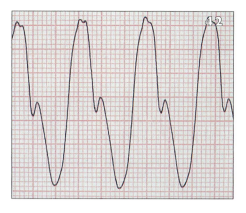

obtained, of which the tracing from lead V5 is shown (**42**, courtesy of Raymond M. Rault). Similar changes were noted in all leads.
i. What are the possible causes of hyperkalaemia in this patient?
ii. Which is most likely?

43 A 56-year-old man complained of severe left flank pain, fever and foul-smelling urine. He had previously had a total cystectomy with a urinary diversion procedure. The patient was febrile, had left flank and upper abdominal tenderness and a right lower quadrant ostomy. Laboratory studies revealed a white blood cell count of 19.5 x 10^9/l and creatinine of 6.0 mg/dl (530 µmol/l). Urinalysis showed many WBCs, occasional RBCs and bacteria. His abdominal

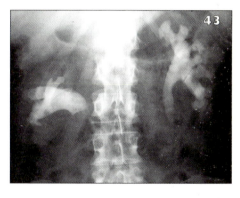

radiograph is shown (**43**). What is the radiologic finding and its aetiology?

44 One month after cadaveric renal transplantation, a patient has an acute rise in serum creatinine. A biopsy was obtained (**44**).
i. What does the biopsy show?
ii. How should this patient be treated?

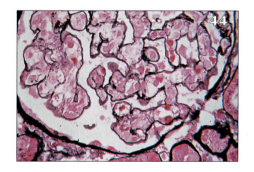

42 i. The possible causes of hyperkalaemia can be divided into four major groups: (a) excess intake of potassium, (b) decreased excretion of potassium, (c) pseudohyperkalaemia and (d) redistribution of potassium from the intracellular space into the vascular space.

ii. In this particular case an excess intake of potassium is unlikely. Decreased excretion is certainly a factor, since the patient is dialysis-dependent and not yet able to excrete a potassium load through the transplanted kidney. Pseudohyperkalaemia occurs when potassium moves out of cells after blood has been drawn, most commonly when red cells haemolyse following venepuncture.

The primary problem in this patient is one of redistribution of potassium between the vascular compartment and the intracellular space in the setting of impaired renal excretion. Potassium is liberated from tissues due to tissue trauma and bleeding during the operation. This potassium is absorbed into the vascular space and normally would re-enter the cells. Potassium entry into cells is augmented by beta$_2$-adrenoreceptors. Activation of these receptors increases adenylate cyclase and Na$^+$,K$^+$-ATPase activity, increasing cellular uptake of potassium. In this case, cellular uptake is inhibited by labetolol, an adrenoreceptor blocking agent with selective alpha$_1$- and non-selective beta-adrenoreceptor blocking action.

Other possible aetiologies of hyperkalaemia from redistribution include hyperglycaemia and metabolic acidosis. Neither of these aetiologies is operative in this case since the patient has a normal plasma glucose and pH.

43 The plain film of his abdomen shows bilateral staghorn calculi. These are most likely struvite, but cystine and uric acid stones can also form staghorn calculi. Struvite stones are composed of magnesium ammonium phosphate and calcium carbonate. Stone formation is favoured in the presence of an alkaline urine and high ammonium concentrations – circumstances seen following urinary tract infections with urease-producing organisms (e.g., *Proteus*). Most struvite stones occur in women because of their higher frequency of urinary tract infections, but they are also seen in association with structural abnormalities of the urinary collecting system that favour recurrent urinary tract infections. Stone growth can be slowed and partial dissolution achieved with the urease inhibitor, acetohydroxamic acid. Unfortunately, this medication is poorly tolerated.

44 i. The biopsy shows an increase in glomerular endothelial cells (i.e., endotheliosis), a finding suggestive of acute vascular rejection. Invasion of the blood vessel walls with inflammatory cells, or vasculitis, may also be seen in acute vascular rejection. Interstitial haemorrhage is another frequent histological finding. Acute cellular rejection, or tubulitis, may also occur in conjunction with acute vascular rejection.
ii. Acute vascular rejection is not likely to respond to a course of high-dose corticosteroids. Therefore, if the risk of additional immunosuppression does not appear to be excessive, treatment with a more potent immunosuppressive agent (e.g., antithymocyte globulin or OKT3) is appropriate.

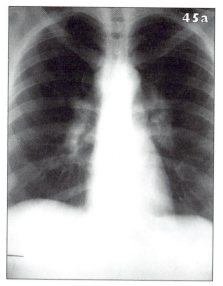
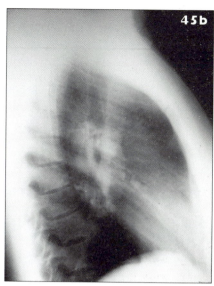

45 A middle-aged black woman is admitted because of confusion. She is mildly orthostatic and has no focal neurological deficits. Laboratory values are serum creatinine 2.2 mg/dl (195 µmol/l), normal electrolytes, serum calcium 13.4 mg/dl (3.35 mmol/l), serum phosphorus 4.4 mg/dl (1.4 mmol/l), and albumin 33 g/l. Chest radiographs are shown (**45a, 45b**).

i. What is the most likely diagnosis?

ii. What is the cause of the hypercalcaemia?

iii. What therapy should you institute?

46 A patient with ADPKD has progressive renal failure and at age 35 years begins maintenance haemodialysis therapy thrice weekly. She desires to have a kidney transplant and her three siblings (20-year-old sister, 28-year-old brother, 35-year-old brother) and parents (57-year-old father, 55-year-old mother) volunteer to be screened as potential donors. Unfortunately, her father has hypertension and her mother's donor work-up reveals bilaterally enlarged cystic kidneys consistent with ADPKD. However, ultrasound screening of her three siblings reveals no detectable renal cysts and they are otherwise healthy. Which family member would you recommend as the kidney donor?

UNIVERSITY OF
SHEFFIELD
LIBRARY

45 i. The combination of hypercalcaemia and bilateral hilar adenopathy is suggestive of sarcoidosis. The differential diagnosis includes tuberculosis, lymphomas and carcinoma. In sarcoidosis, non-caseating granulomas involve multiple organs – lungs, lymph nodes, skin, eye, parotid, liver, etc.

ii. Sarcoidosis commonly causes hypercalciuria, hypercalcaemia and nephrocalcinosis, and can present as an interstitial nephritis with tubular dysfunction. Glomerular involvement is rare. Hypercalcaemia is due to increased conversion of $25(OH)$-D_3 into its active form, $1,25(OH)_2$-D_3 (calcitriol) by sarcoid granulomas, which possess 1-alpha-hydroxylase activity. Calcitriol stimulates bone reabsorption and intestinal absorption of calcium, leading to hypercalcaemia and soft tissue calcifications. Hypercalcaemia lowers PTH, decreasing tubular calcium reabsorption which results in hypercalciuria. Nephrolithiasis occurs in 10% of patients with sarcoidosis. Severe hypercalcaemia may also cause acute renal failure, mediated by renal vasoconstriction (decreased renal blood flow and GFR), and volume depletion resulting from hypercalcaemia-induced nephrogenic diabetes insipidus.

iii. Treatment of hypercalcaemia includes volume repletion and saline diuresis to augment calcium excretion. Corticosteroids are effective in controlling disease activity.

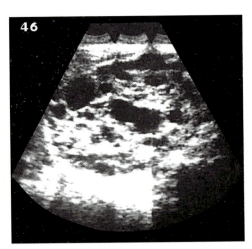

46 Since clinical manifestations of ADPKD are relatively uncommon in children, ultrasound screening is usually not performed before the age of 20 years. In patients with a family history of ADPKD, the standard criteria for a positive radiological screen has been bilateral kidney involvement with a total of at least 3–5 cysts (as shown). A negative renal ultrasound cannot definitively exclude the possibility of ADPKD until the patient is more than 30 years' old. So, the patient's 35-year-old brother would be the first choice for donating a kidney.

47 You are asked to see a 25-year-old man with a 10-year history of ulcerative colitis and recurrent calcium oxalate nephrolithiasis. He has chronic bloody diarrhoea from his ulcerative colitis. The patient avoids milk products, citrus fruit and sources of oxalate. His medications are sulphasalazine and prednisone. His physical examination is unremarkable, except that he appears mildly malnourished. Serum chemistry reveals normal electrolytes, creatinine, calcium, magnesium, uric acid and phosphorus. Two 24-hour urine collections obtained while consuming his usual diet are given (Table).

Test	Usual diet	Usual diet	Units
Volume	3900	3030	ml
pH	6	6	–
Calcium	220	110	mg/day
Phosphorus	860	830	mg/day
Uric acid	600	430	mg/day
Creatinine	1290	1200	mg/day
Urea nitrogen	6900	4700	g/day
Sodium	152	73	mmol/day
Magnesium	2.0	1.3	mEq/day
Oxalate	43	62	mg/day
Citrate	220	170	mg/day

i. What factors contribute to his nephrolithiasis?
ii. What is the significance of the urine magnesium?
iii. What therapy would you prescribe?

48 A 50-year-old man with chronic renal failure secondary to membranous glomerulonephritis received a renal transplant. During the first postoperative 3 months he received three courses of i.v. methylprednisolone for rejection. His blood pressure after 1 year was 210/118 mmHg and there was a loud systolic/diastolic bruit audible over the transplanted kidney. Angiography was therefore performed (**48a**).
i. What does the angiogram show?
ii. What is the the cause of this abnormality?
iii. What other possible diagnosis should have been considered before the angiogram?
iv. How should this be treated?

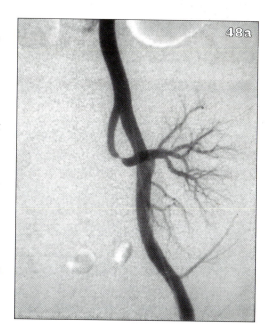

47 i. The primary metabolic abnormalities contributing to his nephrolithiasis are hyperoxaluria and hypocitraturia. Increased luminal bile salt concentrations in inflammatory bowel disease increase bowel oxalate permeability and, by extension, oxaluria. Chronic loss of bicarbonate from diarrhoea can cause metabolic acidosis and decreases urinary citrate excretion.

ii. Hypomagnesiuria occurs in about 5% of stone formers and may contribute to the pathogenesis of calcium oxalate nephrolithiasis. Magnesium can bind to oxalate, thus decreasing its availability to complex with calcium. A good source of dietary magnesium is citrus fruits, which this patient avoided. Magnesium supplements may also be of benefit in patients with hypomagnesiuria and calcium oxalate nephrolithiasis.

iii. Therapy for this man would include increased citrus fruit intake, continued dietary protein (about 1 g protein/kg/day) and sodium restriction, high fluid intake (>2 l/day urine output) and oral potassium citrate. Calcium carbonate could also be used to reduce oxalate absorption and magnesium supplements may improve hypomagnesiuria. Magnesium supplements should be used cautiously since they can cause diarrhoea and worsen hypocitraturia.

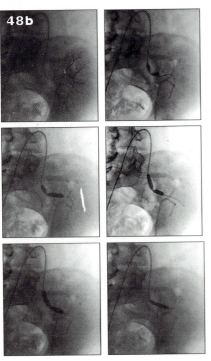

48b

48 i. The angiogram shows stenosis of the transplant renal artery.

ii. Renal artery stenosis occurs in approximately 5% of renal transplant recipients. Four factors may be responsible for its development – rejection of the donor artery, fibrosis at the site of the anastomosis, clamping trauma and atheroma of the recipient's iliac artery.

iii. The other diagnosis that should be considered is an intrarenal arteriovenous fistula. Most commonly this is a complication of renal biopsy. Localised renal ischaemia may be responsible for the increased blood pressure seen in some of these patients. About 75% of fistulae close spontaneously, the remainder may require embolisation.

iv. In transplant renal artery stenosis angioplasty is usually attempted (**48b**) since prolonged renal ischaemia may lead to fibrosis and long-term deterioration in graft function. Surgical repair is associated with an increased risk of graft loss.

49 i. Which of these light microscopy (**49a, 49b, 49c**) patterns is most typical of IgA nephropathy?
ii. What clinical or pathological features at the time of diagnosis predict prognosis in IgA nephropathy?

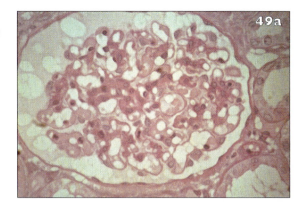

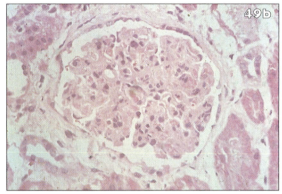

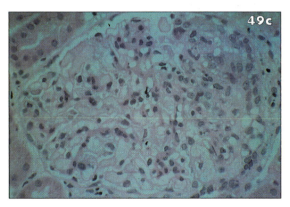

50 A 40-year-old patient with ADPKD presents with fever, acute flank pain and gross haematuria. How would you manage this patient?

49 i. All of them – the light microscopy appearances in IgA nephropathy are variable. This pattern of glomerulonephritis is unique in being defined by the pattern of immune deposits (mesangial IgA) rather than by light microscopy findings.
ii. None are specific to IgA nephropathy – they are the markers of poor prognosis common to any progressive glomerular disease. *Clinical features* are proteinuria, hypertension and renal impairment; a *pathological feature* is glomerular sclerosis.

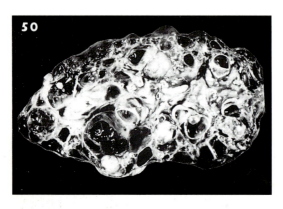

50 Patients with ADPKD may present with fever, haematuria and flank and/or abdominal pain. Often it is difficult clinically to distinguish whether these symptoms are due to urinary tract infection, cyst infection, cyst haemorrhage, nephrolithiasis or, less commonly, renal cancer.

Renal infections occur in 30–50% of ADPKD patients. Not surprisingly, risk factors include female gender and recent urinary tract instrumentation. Pyuria can be found in up to 45% of uninfected ADPKD patients. However, white cell casts and positive urine cultures suggest acute pyelonephritis, while focal areas of flank or abdominal tenderness may be seen with intracystic infections. Occasionally, perinephric abscess or bacteraemia may complicate the course. Radiological studies (ultrasound, CT, IVP, nuclear imaging) usually cannot distinguish renal infection from cyst haemorrhage, but may be helpful in ruling out an obstructing stone. In acute pyelonephritis, typical antimicrobial regimens such as ampicillin, a cephalosporin or an aminoglycoside (dose adjusted for the level of renal insufficiency) are usually efficacious. However, for intracystic infections, therapy with lipid-soluble antibiotics (e.g., chloramphenicol, ciprofloxacin, trimethoprim–sulphamethoxazole) may be required for 4–6 weeks in order to eradicate the infection. Relapse of cyst infections may necessitate 2–3 months of antimicrobial treatment. Radiographic localisation of the infected cyst is often impossible, making percutaneous drainage a rare therapeutic option. Surgical nephrectomy in ADPKD (**50**) is reserved for renal transplant candidates with a history of recurrent, refractory or complicated renal infections.

51 A patient with AIDS has been treated for several weeks for a CMV infection. The patient is noted to have a sudden deterioration in mental status and laboratory data are: serum Na$^+$ 118 mmol/l, serum K$^+$ 6.7 mmol/l, serum Cl$^-$ 84 mmol/l, serum HCO$_3^-$ 20 mmol/l, BUN 22 mg/dl (7.9 mmol/l), creatinine 1.8 mg/dl (160 μmol/l) and glucose 42 mg/dl (2.3 mmol/l). The patient's blood pressure is 100/60 mmHg and he is orthostatic. Which of the following is the most likely explanation for these results?
i. Acute hypothyroidism.
ii. Type IV RTA.
iii. Acute adrenal insufficiency.
iv. CNS lesion with panhypopituitary state.

52 An 80-year-old man, treated for hypertension with a thiazide diuretic, develops diarrhoea and abdominal pain. He buys an 'over the counter' analgesic from his pharmacy. After taking three tablets daily for 4 days, his diarrhoea and abdominal pain resolve, but he now complains of vomiting, muscle weakness and palpitations. He is admitted to hospital where his blood pressure is 120/70 mmHg lying and 90/60 mmHg standing; his neck veins are not visible and skin turgor is decreased. An ECG shows peaked T waves in the precordial leads. The serum sodium is 140 mmol/l, urea 70 mg/dl (25 mmol/l), creatinine 2.4 mg/dl (210 μmol/l) and potassium 7.2 mmol/l. Urinalysis shows protein+

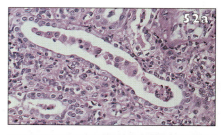

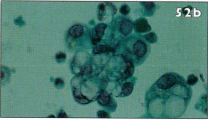

and microscopy of the urine sediment shows occasional renal tubular cells and many granular casts. A renal biopsy is shown (**52a**), as is the urine cytology (**52b**).
i. What is your clinical diagnosis?
ii. Why is the serum potassium elevated?
iii. Interpret the renal biopsy.

53 A 45-year-old man with human immunodeficiency virus infection is admitted with a productive cough and dyspnoea. Physical examination showed a temperature of 37.5°C, respiratory rate of 24 breaths per minute, blood pressure of 110/70 mmHg and a pulse of 110 b.p.m. Chest examination revealed a bilateral basilar rales and a chest radiograph showed diffuse infiltrates. Serum electrolytes, blood urea nitrogen and creatinine are normal. Sputum cultures reveal *Pneumocystis carinii* and therapy is initiated with trimethoprim (20 mg/kg/day) and sulphamethoxazole (100 mg/kg/day). The patient improves but on the ninth day of therapy, the serum potassium is noted to have risen from its previously normal value of 4.1 to 6.0 mmol/l. What is the most likely cause of the patient's hyperkalaemia?

51 iii. Adrenalitis is a fairly common sequela of CMV infection in patients with AIDS. The constellation of hyponatraemia, hyperkalaemia, metabolic acidosis, hypoglycaemia and hypotension is almost diagnostic. Hyperkalaemia in these patients is probably secondary to hypoaldosteronism. The hyponatraemia seen in adrenal insufficiency appears to be multifactorial. Experimentally, glucocorticoids appear to have an ADH-independent effect on water conservation. The hypotension resulting from sodium wasting also results in volume-mediated (non-osmotic) ADH release. Hypothyroidism can produce hyponatraemia, but not hyperkalaemia. A type IV RTA is usually associated with normal or elevated blood pressure and not with hyponatraemia or hypoglycaemia. A panhypopituitary state could produce these clinical findings, but is rare in this clinical setting. However, it should probably be evaluated after a cortisol level has been obtained and glucocorticoid replacement instituted.

52 i. This patient has ATN secondary to non-steroidal anti-inflammatory drugs (NSAIDs). Acute renal failure has become an increasing problem as NSAIDs have become one of the most commonly used medications, particulary in the elderly. Risk factors for NSAID-induced acute renal failure include old age and dehydration, here resulting from the simultaneous use of diuretics and development of diarrhoea.
ii. NSAIDs can cause hyperkalaemia by inhibiting prostaglandin-mediated renin release, leading to a hyporeninaemic hypoaldosteronism. The mechanism for acute renal failure from NSAIDs is ischaemic damage to oxygen-demanding tubules secondary to vasoconstriction of the afferent arteriole where prostaglandins have a vasodilatory action.
iii. The urine cytology (52b) shows renal tubular epithelial cells. These are frequently seen in ATN, along with tubular cell and granular casts. The renal biopsy (52a) shows a renal tubular cell cast within the lumen of a tubule.

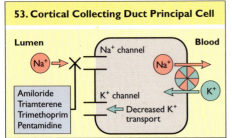

53. Cortical Collecting Duct Principal Cell

53 Elevations of serum potassium are frequently seen in AIDS patients receiving high-dose trimethoprim–sulphamethoxazole therapy for *Pneumocystis carinii* pneumonia. Trimethoprim is structurally related to the potassium-sparing diuretics, triamterene and amiloride, which can induce hyperkalaemia by interfering with renal potassium excretion. All of these agents appear to inhibit sodium transport by blocking luminal sodium channels in the principal cells of the cortical collecting duct (53). Inhibition of sodium entry into these cells decreases the lumen negative potential difference across the membrane which, in turn, reduces the electrical gradient that favours passive potassium secretion.

Serum potassium should be closely monitored in patients with AIDS who receive high-dose trimethoprim therapy. A similar concern is warranted for patients with renal insufficiency who receive this drug.

54 i. Describe the two CAPD catheters shown in 54.
ii. What are the putative advantages of the lower catheter?

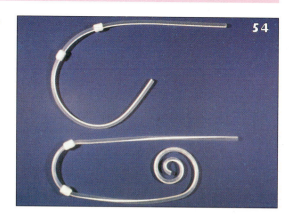

55 i. What extrarenal manifestation of ADPKD is shown on this CT scan (55)?
ii. What are the other common extrarenal manifestations of ADPKD?

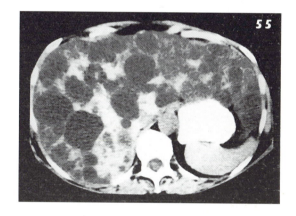

56 This 39-year-old man was referred after his family physician found him to have an elevated serum creatinine when he presented with general malaise.
i. What abnormality is shown in 56?
ii. What investigations would you undertake to identify the primary cause of the renal impairment?

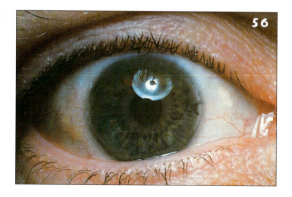

54 i. Above is a conventional double cuff Tenckhoff catheter; below is a curled tip, swan neck, double cuff catheter.
ii. Nearly all CAPD catheters have two cuffs as these have better long-term survival than single cuff catheters. Coiling of the tip into a curved form is designed to reduce the incidence of catheter migration and omental obstruction. The swan neck between the two cuffs is designed to ensure that the catheter exits the skin in a caudal direction, facilitating drainage and reducing the likelihood of exit site infection. The potential benefits of different CAPD catheter designs have in general not been tested in controlled prospective studies

55 i. The CT scan shows hepatic cysts. The prevalence increases from 10% in ADPKD patients <30 years to more than 40% in patients >60 years of age. Usually hepatic cysts are asymptomatic, but occasionally they may become infected or enlarge, resulting in pain. Congenital hepatic fibrosis is only rarely seen in ADPKD.
ii. In addition to kidney involvement, patients with ADPKD frequently have abnormalities involving other organ systems. The nature of these abnormalities suggests that a common defect in epithelial and/or connective tissue expression is responsible for the disease manifestations of ADPKD.

Colonic diverticuli and inguinal and umbilical hernias appear with increased frequency in the ADPKD population. Clinical presentations include abdominal pain, alterations in bowel habits and lower gastrointestinal bleeding. The incidence of diverticular disease is even higher in patients with ADPKD who receive maintenance dialysis.

Transthoracic echocardiography detects valvular heart disease (usually mitral valve prolapse or aortic regurgitation) in 25% of patients with ADPKD. Most valvular lesions are asymptomatic, but if heard on auscultation patients should receive antibiotic prophylaxis.

Cerebral aneurysms occur in 10–22% of ADPKD patients. The incidence increases from 4% in young adults to 10% in older adults. Kindreds with a family history of cerebral aneurysms or intracerebral haemorrhage are at greatest risk. In one study of ADPKD patients with cerebral aneurysms, 50% had normal renal function (involvement of the middle cerebral artery predominated), 31% had multiple aneurysms and in 48% death or severe disability ensued. Routine screening with CT or MRI is usually reserved for high-risk patients; i.e. those with a family history of subarachnoid haemorrhage, severe headaches or previous aneurysmal rupture or high-risk occupations where loss of consciousness is undesirable. Surgery is reserved for patients with symptomatic aneurysms or aneurysms >10 mm in diameter.

56 i. The abnormality shown is a band keratopathy due to hypercalcaemia.
ii. Further investigations to elucidate the cause of the hypercalcaemia would include measurement of serum iPTH to exclude hyperparathyroidism, a chest radiograph to exclude hilar lymphadenopathy due to sarcoidosis, measurement of serum immunoglobulins and protein electrophoresis to exclude myeloma.

57 A young black man presents with
gross haematuria, flank pain and
moderate renal insufficiency. A
retrograde pyelogram is performed
(57).
i. What is the diagnosis?
ii. What additional diagnostic studies
would you perform?

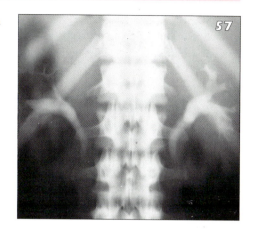

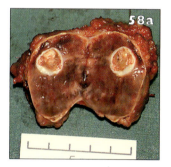

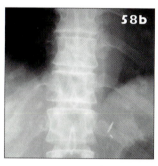

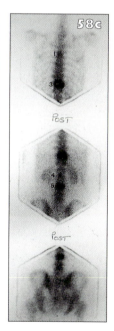

58 A 56-year-old woman presented with headache and
postural 'dizziness'. Blood pressure was 182/114 mmHg
sitting and 134/80 mmHg standing. Investigations showed a
phaeochromocytoma in the right adrenal gland which was
removed (58a). A year later she complained of back pain, so
a radiograph of the spine (58b) and a bone scan (58c) were
obtained.
i. What is the likely cause of the postural hypotension?
ii. What do the radiograph of the spine and bone scan show?
iii. What other investigations would you undertake?

57 i. The diagnosis is papillary necrosis. The urographic findings associated with papillary necrosis include caliceal deformity with clubbing. Early urographic signs include parallel streaks of contrast originating at the papilla and extending towards the cortex, indicating early papillary detachment. In more advanced stages, the streaks become confluent giving the appearance of a 'lobster claw', which may extend around the papilla to produce the classic 'ring' sign. Occasionally, the papilla may calcify, seen as small calcified deposits on the radiograph. Filling defects along the ureter may represent sloughed papillae.

ii. The imaging procedure of choice is an IVP with tomograms. Patients with renal insufficiency may require retrograde studies. Renal ultrasound and CT scan are not as sensitive as the IVP, but may detect advanced papillary necrosis, especially when associated with calcifications. As shown here, the disease process is not uniform; some papillae may be severely damaged, while others are spared.

Papillary necrosis is common in patients with sickle cell haemoglobinopathies (both sickle cell disease and trait), occurring in up to 40% of patients. It typically occurs in young adults, in contrast to papillary necrosis associated with other diseases which present in older adults. A haemoglobin electrophoresis should be performed in patients of African or Mediterranean descent who present with symptoms suggestive of papillary necrosis. Haematuria, sometimes associated with flank pain, is the presenting symptom, and usually responds to rest and hydration. The prognosis of papillary necrosis in sickle cell disease is good, as patients do not usually progress to end-stage renal failure. Other causes of papillary necrosis include diabetes mellitus, obstructive uropathy, pyelonephritis and analgesic abuse.

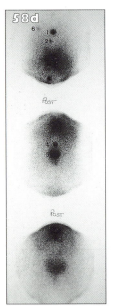

58 i. Postural hypotension is a recognised feature of phaeochromocytoma. It is thought to be due to down regulation of α-receptors by high circulating catecholamine levels. Treatment with α-blockers may also cause postural hypotension.

ii. The radiograph of the spine shows lytic lesions and the bone scan multiple 'hot' spots.

iii. Of phaeochromocytoma, 10% are malignant. To determine whether these lesions are metastases, measurement of urinary catecholamines and a radiolabelled MIBG (metaiodobenzylguanidine) scan (**58d**) should be undertaken. MIBG is taken up specifically by cells synthesising catecholamines. There is no proven treatment for metastatic phaeochromocytoma. Standard practice is to block the action of adrenaline (epinephrine) and noradrenaline (norepinephrine) with phenoxybenzamine and a beta-blocker. There are reports of the use of high dose radioactive MIBG; this patient received this therapy and has remained well for 8 years.

59 This 42-year-old black male renal transplant recipient complained of sore gums and bleeding after brushing his teeth (59). He had been receiving maintenance immunosuppression with prednisone, cyclosporin and azathioprine for 2 years.
i. What is the cause?
ii. What is the therapy?

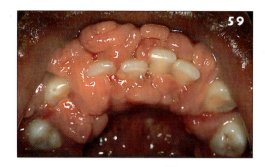

60 The investigation shown in 60 has been undertaken in a child.
i. What is the study?
ii. What does it show?

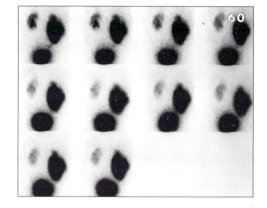

61 A renal transplant patient developed progressive nocturia and polyuria. An ultrasound revealed hydronephrosis without any adjacent fluid collections. A diagnostic study was then performed (61). What does it show?

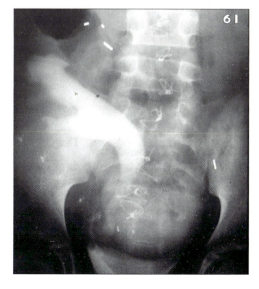

59 i. The patient is exhibiting advanced gingival hypertrophy resulting from chronic administration of CSA. The mechanism is poorly understood, but is aggravated by poor dentition and calcium channel blockers.
ii. Therapy involves a programme of oral hygiene, including frequent brushing with a baking soda-based toothpaste, dental flossing and periodontal rinses. In more advanced cases, such as this one, gingivectomy or surgical debridement may be necessary. There have been reports of improvements in response to a course of antibiotics, such as metronidazole. Other agents which may cause gingival hyperplasia, such as calcium channel blockers, should be discontinued if possible. Reducing the cyclosporin dosage generally does little more than expose the patient to an increased risk of graft loss. Conversion to tacrolimus (FK506) may be considered, as this agent may provide comparable immunosuppression without this particular side-effect.

60 i. This is a MAG3 furosemide renogram.
ii. It shows a ureteropelvic junction obstruction. Children with hydronephrosis seldom present with flank pain, urinary tract infection or haematuria. When asymptomatic hydronephrosis is discovered on renal ultrasound, it is important to ascertain whether the dilatation of the collecting system represents obstruction or simply an ectatic collecting system. Therefore, more attention is being focussed on quantitating renal function, with nuclear renography being an increasingly popular modality. MAG3 is the radioisotope of choice, with furosemide administered to promote urine flow and an indwelling catheter placed to ensure bladder drainage. Despite its popularity, it should be appreciated that nuclear renography is fraught with pitfalls and its utility is operator-dependent. Ultrasonography is the imaging procedure of choice for the initial evaluation of renal anatomy.

The Whitaker study has been suggested as the gold standard for diagnosing obstruction. The main problem with this test lies in the non-physiological conditions under which it is performed. It requires percutaneous placement of a nephrostomy tube and maintenance of urine flow rates of at least 10 ml per minute. These high flow rates are certainly inappropriate for a neonate weighing 10 kg who would normally have urine flow rates of 3–5 ml/kg/h. It is important to obtain a VCUG to determine whether reflux is also present.

61 The contrast study demonstrates that the patient has partial obstruction of the distal ureter. The cause was secondary to ureteral ischaemia. The vascular supply to the distal ureter may be compromised during organ procurement, and in time ischaemia may result in scarring, stricture and/or vesicocritical reflux. Therapeutic options include stenting the ureteral vesicle junction for prolonged periods if the ureter is viable. Alternatively, it may be necessary to remove the involved segment and reattach the ureter to the bladder, or create an anastomosis with the ipsilateral native ureter to re-establish a proper urinary conduit.

62 A 50-year-old woman with ESRD secondary to hypertension undergoes coronary artery bypass surgery for unstable angina. Her operative course is uncomplicated and during the post-operative period she resumes her regular dialysis treatments and medications. Post-operatively, meperidine (pethidine) hydrochloride 50 mg is administered intramuscularly every 4 hours for pain. Dialysis therapy is uneventful with excellent clearance and blood pressure control. On the fourth post-operative day the patient develops myoclonus and has a grand-mal seizure. A CT scan of the brain shows no evidence of bleeding or cerebral infarction. Neurology is consulted and ascribes the seizures and myoclonus to toxic–metabolic disturbances related to inadequate dialysis.

i. What other aetiologies for seizures should be considered in this patient?
ii. How could this problem have been avoided?

63 A middle-aged woman is admitted because of nephrotic syndrome and mild renal insufficiency. A kidney biopsy was performed (63a, haematoxylin and eosin; 63b, kappa IgA antibody immunofluorescence; 63c, EM; courtesy of R. Hennigar, MD, and A. Someren, MD). What is the differential diagnosis?

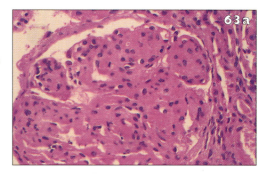

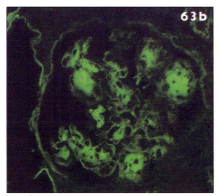

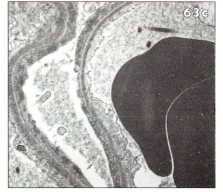

62 i. Drugs must always be considered as a possible cause of altered CNS function in patients with impaired renal function. Meperidine is primarily metabolised in the liver by hydrolysis to meperidinic acid followed by conjugation with glucuronic acid. Meperidine may also undergo N-demethylation to normeperidine, which is excreted primarily in the urine. Normeperidine is a pharmacologically active metabolite, with about 50% of the analgesic activity of meperidine but twice the CNS stimulation of the parent drug. Accumulation of normeperidine results in toxic side effects due to CNS stimulation, including agitation, tremor, twitching, myoclonus and seizures.
ii. Prolonged administration of meperidine in patients with renal insufficiency should be avoided because of the decreased renal excretion of normeperidine. When narcotic analgesia is needed for patients with decreased renal function, morphine sulphate or hydromorphine hydrochloride is recommended. Narcotic-induced side effects can be minimised by using the smallest effective doses of these analgesics in patients with renal failure.

63 63a shows mesangial expansion with nodular glomerulosclerosis (reminiscent of Kimmelstiel–Wilson diabetic nodules) and glomerular basement membrane thickening. Based on light microscopy, the differential diagnosis includes diabetic glomerulosclerosis and light chain nephropathy. The final diagnosis will depend on the results of immunofluorescence and EM studies. In diabetes, a non-specific trapping of circulating proteins is seen on immunofluorescence, and on EM the glomerular basement membrane is diffusely, homogeneously thickened. In light chain nephropathy, a monoclonal protein is demonstrated by immunofluorescence (**63b**), and on EM granular electron dense deposits are present along the subendothelial aspect of the glomerular basement membrane. Subepithelial deposits may also present, as in **63c**. The combination of light microscopy, immunofluorescence and EM findings are diagnostic of light chain nephropathy.

Light chain nephropathy is one of the monoclonal immunoglobulin deposition diseases (MIDD), comprising light and heavy chain nephropathies. It is usually associated with plasma cell dyscrasias or multiple myeloma. In the majority of cases the deposits include kappa light chains. Light chain glomerulopathy is a multisystem disease, with deposits in the liver, heart, skin, gastrointestinal tract, etc. Chemotherapy, with monthly cycles of prednisone and melphalan, is the treatment of choice. Renal prognosis is determined by the level of renal function at presentation. Most patients with serum creatinine >4 mg/dl (350 µmol/l) will progress to ESRD despite therapy, whereas for those patients with more preserved function, treatment may decrease proteinuria and stabilise renal function.

64 A 19-year-old man who had been receiving home haemodialysis for over a decade slowly developed this lesion (64a) on his right thumb. The mass was non-tender, had a smooth surface and a solid consistency.
i. What is this abnormality?
ii. What treatment options are available?

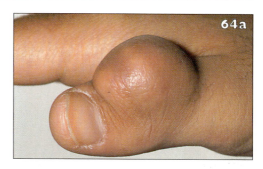

65 Shown here are the CT scan of the kidneys (65a) and a renal arteriogram (65b) of a 34-year-old woman who presented with general malaise and acute renal failure.
i. What does the CT scan (65a) show?
ii. What does the renal arteriogram (65b) show?
iii. What is the likely diagnosis and what other investigation would you undertake to confirm this?

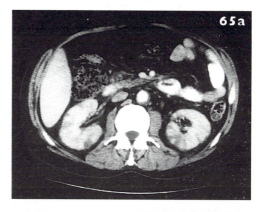

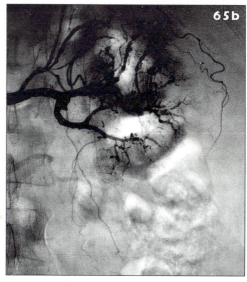

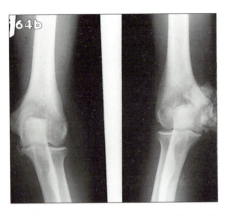

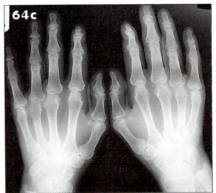

64 i. The mass on the patient's thumb is caused by tumoral (metastatic) calcification. This variety of soft-tissue calcification in long-term dialysis patients is typically distributed in periarticular locations. The deposits can become sizeable (**64b**) and can significantly restrict joint movements. The lesions are generally painless, but may become secondarily infected. These calcium deposits consist of carbonate-containing apatite, similar to that found in bone.

Vascular calcification (see radial artery calcification in **64c**) has a similar composition, and is seen both in an intimal and a medial distribution. Intimal calcification, seen typically in the aorta and large arteries, may aggravate pre-existing atheromatous lesions and contribute to ischaemia. Medial calcification involves medium-size vessels and may cause the syndrome of calciphylaxis, characterised by progressive, gangrenous ulceration of the skin of digits, ankles, thighs and buttocks.

ii. The aetiology of both tumoral and vascular calcification is uncertain, but as with visceral calcification (see **81**) a high calcium:phosphate ratio blood product appears pivotal in the genesis of these complications. Treatment should be preventative. Established lesions often prove refractory to treatment. Prolonged normalisation of biochemistry, even after parathyroidectomy and/or renal transplantation, often fails to mobilise tumoral and vascular calcium deposits. Surgical removal of tumoral deposits may be necessary to improve joint function or to eradicate secondary infection, which may be life-threatening. Parathyroidectomy is the treatment of choice for the rare syndrome of calciphylaxis.

65 i. The CT scan (**65a**) shows multiple, small 'wedge-shaped' infarcts in the kidneys. These could be due to a vasculitis, such as Wegener's granulomatosis, polyarterits nodosa or bacterial endocarditis.

ii. The renal arteriogram (**65b**) shows multiple small aneurysms.

iii. The likely diagnosis is polyarteritis nodosa – the presence of pANCA in a significant titre would confirm this.

66 An 83-year-old woman was found collapsed on her kitchen floor. Clinical examination suggested that she had suffered a cerebrovascular accident. Subsequent investigations revealed acute renal failure. Here is shown the light microscopy of her centrifuged urine sediment (66).
i. What is the likely cause of her acute renal failure?
ii. What other investigations should be done to confirm the diagnosis?

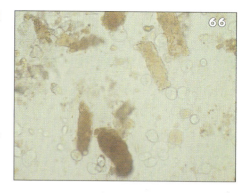

67 A 67-year-old retired farmer presents with a facial lesion (67) which he has had for the previous 4 months. He frequently cuts it after shaving and has recently noted that it is taking longer for bleeding to cease. For the past 10 years he has had excellent renal allograft function on a stable regimen of prednisone, azathioprine and cyclosporin.
i. What is the lesion?
ii. What is the most appropriate therapy?

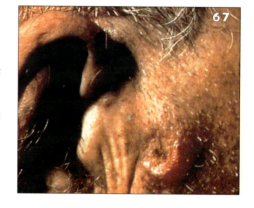

68 i. What is the diagnosis and most likely aetiology for the condition shown in 68?
ii. What is the correct treatment in this case?

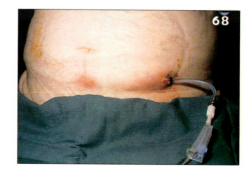

66 i. The urine microscopy demonstrates numerous granular casts, suggesting a renal parenchymal cause for the acute renal failure. However, these casts have a typical golden yellow colour. In this patient the cast pigmentation was due to myoglobulinuria, secondary to acute rhabdomyolysis resulting from prolonged muscle pressure while the patient was collapsed on her kitchen floor. Other causes of golden pigmentation of urinary casts are haemoglobinuria and jaundice.
ii. Acute rhabdomyolysis and acute haemoglobinaemia may be differentiated at the bedside. A blood sample is left to sediment and the plasma inspected. The plasma will remain pink in haemoglobinaemia, but is of normal colour in acute rhabdomyolysis. The diagnosis of acute rhabdomyolysis is confirmed by the finding of elevated plasma levels of muscle enzymes [typically creatine phosphokinase (CPK)], and the measurement of urinary myoglobin.

67 i. The differential diagnosis of a skin lesion such as this must include squamous cell carcinoma until proven otherwise. Squamous cell carcinomas are seen with increased frequency in the transplant population (especially in older patients) and, in contrast to the general population, the prevalence is twice that of the generally less aggressive basal cell carcinoma. Skin cancers are the most common malignancies in the transplant population and increase in frequency with time. Risk factors include chronic and excessive ultraviolet light exposure (including early childhood sunburns), fair complexion, premalignant lesions and type and/or degree of immunosuppression. In Australian renal transplant recipients, there is an extraordinary preponderance of these risk factors leading to a 100-fold risk increase.
ii. Excisional biopsy is appropriate in this case. For patients with rapid development of squamous cell carcinoma following transplantation, or in those experiencing frequent recurrences, tapering of the immunosuppressive regimen is appropriate. In addition, there may be a benefit in using retinoid preparations to reduce recurrences. More aggressive lesions, such as those which are deeply invasive or metastatic, may require more drastic measures, including withdrawal of immunosuppression, radiation therapy or chemotherapy.

68 i. This patient has a severe catheter exit-site infection extending along the subcutaneous tunnel. The infecting organism is probably *Staphylococcus aureus* – *Pseudomonas* would be a less likely possibility. Staphylococcal infections usually occur at the time of catheter insertion and nasal carriers of *S. aureus* are at increased risk. Exit infection may be prevented in some patients by the use of perioperative anti-staphylococcal antibiotic therapy or by eradication of nasal staphylococcal carriage.
ii. The correct treatment in this case is prompt removal of the catheter in addition to appropriate parenteral antibiotic therapy. Some might advocate replacing the catheter on the other side of the abdomen at the same operation, but most would defer this for 2–4 weeks until the initial infection has cleared fully.

69 A 17-year-old patient with type I insulin-dependent diabetes mellitus is seen in the emergency department. Laboratory data are as follows: serum Na^+ 130 mmol/l, serum K^+ 6.1 mmol/l, serum Cl^- 90 mmol/l, serum HCO_3^- 14 mmol/l, BUN 17 mg/dl (6.1 mmol/l), creatinine 1.5 mg/dl (133 μmol/l) and glucose 480 mg/dl (27 mmol/l). Serum ketones are positive. Blood pressure is 120/80 mmHg and the patient is orthostatic. Which of the following best explains this patient's hyperkalaemia?
i. Metabolic acidosis.
ii. Hyperosmolarity.
iii. Insulinopenia.
iv. Adrenal insufficiency.

70 A 60-year-old obese woman with severe osteo-arthritis is started on a NSAID. After 2 months she returns to her physician complaining of swelling of both legs. Her serum creatinine is 2.9 mg/dl (260 μmol/l), serum albumin 20 g/l, and a 24-hour urine collection contains 11 g of protein. Urinalysis reveals protein 3+, and urine microscopy fine and coarsely granulated casts.
i. What is the clinical diagnosis?
ii. What does the renal biopsy show (70a, 70b)?

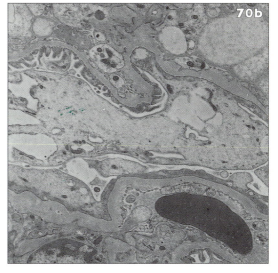

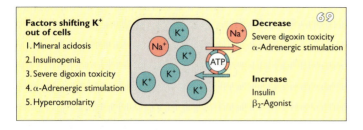

Factors shifting K$^+$ out of cells		Decrease	69
1. Mineral acidosis		Severe digoxin toxicity	
2. Insulinopenia		α-Adrenergic stimulation	
3. Severe digoxin toxicity			
4. α-Adrenergic stimulation		**Increase**	
5. Hyperosmolarity		Insulin	
		β_2-Agonist	

69 ii, iii. In diabetic ketoacidosis, patients often present with hyperkalaemia. Interestingly, the total body potassium of these patients may actually be decreased secondary to urinary losses from the osmotic diuresis, which is almost always present. Extracellular hyperosmolarity will draw potassium-rich fluid out of the intracellular space to produce an increase in serum potassium. The primary factor controlling intracellular potassium concentration is the Na$^+$/K$^+$-ATP-ase (see **69**). Insulin is an important regulator of Na$^+$/K$^+$-ATP-ase and the combination of hyperosmolarity and insulinopenia are sufficient to explain the hyperkalaemia seen in diabetic ketoacidosis. While mineral acidosis may shift potassium out of cells, organic acidosis, e.g., lactic and ketoacidosis, does not. Adrenal insufficiency is not likely given the clinical scenario and the hyponatraemia in this case is largely due to the intra- to extra-cellular movement of water resulting from hyperglycaemia.

70 i. The presence of oedema, hypoalbuminaemia and proteinuria exceeding 3.5 g/day is diagnostic of the nephrotic syndrome. The various causes of this disorder are discussed elsewhere, but the temporal relationship makes NSAIDs a prime suspect in this case.
ii. The renal biopsy shows severe interstitial inflammation (**70a**) with fusion of the foot processes on electron microscopy (**70b**). In NSAID-induced nephrosis the renal histology typically shows a normal glomerular structure by light microscopy, with fusion of the foot processes on electron microscopy, features similar to idiopathic minimal change disease. However, in contrast to idiopathic minimal change disease, NSAID-induced nephrosis is associated with a prominent mononuclear interstitial infiltrate.

71 A 38-year-old woman with known bilateral renal artery stenosis not amenable to surgery or angioplasty has hypertension which is resistant to treatment with beta-blockers, calcium channel blockers and diuretics. She is prescribed minoxidil which results in good control of blood pressure.

i. Describe her facial appearance (71).

ii. What are the side effects of minoxidil and what are the mechanisms through which they occur?

iii. What is the place of minoxidil in the management of hypertension?

iv. Which other drugs might have been tried before minoxidil?

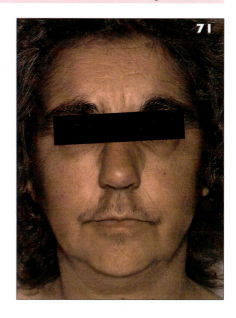

72 An elderly diabetic presents with fever, hypotension, flank pain and obtundation. Urine and blood grew *Escherichia coli*. Despite aggressive management, the patient died. A kidney specimen at autopsy is shown in 72 (Courtesy of K. Hewan-Lowe, MD). What is the pathological diagnosis?

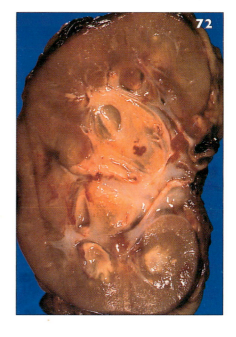

71 i. There is an increase in facial hair affecting the upper lip, chin, neck, forehead and cheeks.

ii. Minoxidil increases hair growth by increasing skin blood flow through its powerful vasodilatory action. The hair growth resolves on withdrawal of the drug. Minoxidil may also cause profound fluid retention and loop diuretics may be necessary to counteract this. ST depression and T wave inversion may be seen when minoxidil is first introduced, due to reflex sympathetic stimulation induced by the vasodilatation. Pericardial effusion has been reported but the mechanism is not known.

iii. Minoxidil is usually reserved for resistant hypertension. However, it does not cause impotence and can be used in patients who experience this side effect with other agents.

iv. The selective alpha-1 blockers doxazosin or methyldopa might have been used before minoxidil.

72 The pathology specimen revealed acute, diffuse inflammatory changes of the kidney (acute pyelonephritis) and the presence of necrotic papillae in the lower pole. Intact papillae are seen at the upper pole.

Diseases associated with papillary necrosis include diabetes mellitus, acute pyelonephritis, analgesic nephropathy, sickle cell anaemia, obstructive uropathy and acute transplant rejection. In diabetes, the incidence of papillary necrosis is 10-fold greater than seen in the general population. Bacterial pyelonephritis is almost always present and may contribute to papillary necrosis. Obstructive uropathy, analgesics and NSAIDs are also predisposing factors for papillary necrosis in diabetes. The pathogenesis involves vascular insufficiency caused by microvascular occlusion of the renal medullary circulation, resulting in decreased blood flow and medullary hypoxia. Blood flow may also be compromised by interstitial oedema (as in acute pyelonephritis), or by the back pressure and renal haemodynamic changes associated with obstructive uropathy. NSAIDs may cause papillary necrosis by blocking vasodilatory prostaglandin production, thus reducing medullary blood flow. Papillary necrosis usually presents with flank pain, fever, chills, dysuria and haematuria, mimicking renal colic. Rarely, a necrosed papillae may be recovered in the urine. Radiological findings include papillary deformities and the presence of a 'ring' sign on an IVP. Therapy is directed at the underlying cause, i.e., treatment of the UTI, relief of obstruction, etc. Nephrotoxic drugs, especially NSAIDs, should be avoided.

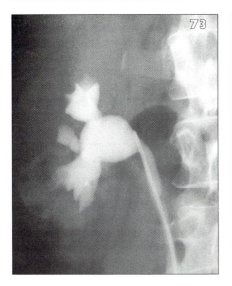

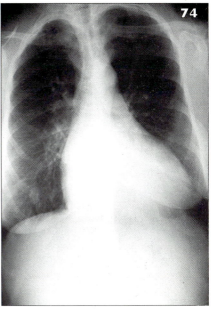

73 A 37-year-old man presented with a 3-month history of low-grade fevers, general malaise, urinary urgency and dysuria, but no other medical problems; his only medication was the antibiotic prescribed for his chronic 'urinary tract infection'. His temperature was 37.7°C, a chest examination revealed crackles in the left apex, abdominal examination was normal and there was no CVA tenderness. His urinalysis showed 20–30 WBCs and 5–10 RBCs per high power field. A urine culture was negative on two occasions and his chest radiograph revealed a left upper lobe infiltrate. A retrograde pyelogram (73) and special urine cultures were performed. What is the aetiology of his pyuria?

74 Three months after renal transplantation, this 37-year-old construction worker had a routine chest radiograph (74). What is the differential diagnosis?

75 The Table gives analyses for three patients with glomerulonephritis. What diagnosis should be considered in each case?

Patient	Serum C3 (mg/dl)	Serum C4 (mg/dl)
Case 1	44	12
Case 2	135	9
Case 3	37	51
Reference ranges	85–190	20–80

73 The pyelogram shows multiple amorphous renal parenchymal calcifications consistent with renal tuberculosis. This diagnosis is further supported by the low-grade fever, constitutional symptoms and sterile pyuria. Renal tuberculosis results from haematogenous spread of *M. tuberculosis*. Once the kidney is seeded, granulomas can rupture into tubules and cause pyuria. Routine cultures are usually negative and urine must be sent specifically for AFB cultures. Sensitivity is improved by collecting three or more morning first-void specimens, since only 30–40% of urine cultures are positive. Patients can present with dysuria, frequency, nocturia, urgency, haematuria and back, flank or abdominal pain. They frequently do not have constitutional symptoms. Hypertension is an uncommon complication of renal tuberculosis. The intravenous pyelogram may be normal, but often shows calyceal blunting, papillary necrosis, scarring and parenchymal calcifications. Other sources of sterile pyuria include interstitial nephritis, urethritis and, rarely, glomerulonephritis.

74 The differential diagnosis of a single, asymptomatic pulmonary nodule is similar to that for multiple pulmonary nodules (see **211**). This patient had pulmonary aspergillosis, probably resulting from inhalation of these common soil spores while working on construction sites. Itraconazole was given, and there was complete resolution of the nodule. Immunosuppression was continued along with the itraconazole, and graft function was preserved. This case also illustrates the potential value of routine screening in populations with a high incidence of disease.

75 Case 1: *Active lupus nephritis*. Depression of both C3 and C4 indicates classic pathway complement activation, which is characteristic of active systemic lupus. Case 2: *Inactive systemic lupus*. In inactive lupus C4 may remain low even if C3 returns to normal, since a genetic trait that results in low C4 production (C4 null allele) is associated with lupus.
Case 3. If C3 is low but C4 normal, this suggests alternative pathway complement activation. This occurs in nephritis associated with endocarditis, post-infectious glomerulonephritis, glomerulonephritis associated with mixed essential cryoglobulinaemia, and mesangiocapillary glomerulonephritis (in the last case C3 activation is provoked by C3 nephritic factor, an autoantibody which stabilises C3 convertase).

76 A 65-year-old woman is admitted with a 2-day history of fever, rigors, dysuria and right flank pain. Serum creatinine on admission is 1 mg/dl (90 µmol/l). Therapy is instituted with intravenous gentamicin 80 mg every 8 hours and intravenous fluids. Blood and urine cultures grow *Pseudomonas aeruginosa* sensitive only to gentamicin and tobramycin.

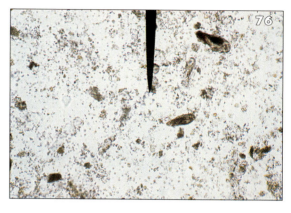

Gentamicin therapy is continued and the patient improves. On the third hospital day serum creatinine is 0.9 mg/dl (80 µmol/l), but on day seven it is 3.1 mg/dl (270 µmol/l). Urine microscopy shows numerous granular casts (**76**, courtesy of Arthur Greenberg). Urine sodium is 45 mmol/l with a fractional excretion of sodium (FE_{Na}) of 2.0%.
i. What is the most likely cause of the acute renal failure in this patient?
ii. How could renal failure have been avoided?

77 i. What is the likely cause of renal failure in this 20-year-old man with spina bifida (**76**)?
ii. What are the relative and absolute contraindications to peritoneal dialysis in such a case?

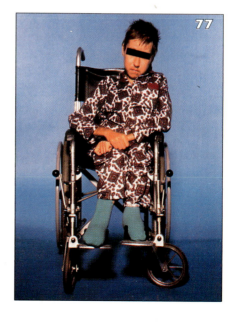

76 i. If the patient's hypotension had persisted after admission, pre-renal acute renal failure could develop, eventually leading to ischaemic ATN. The rapid normalisation of blood pressure, maintenance of good urine output, high urine sodium and FE_{Na} argue against pre-renal causes. ATN due to the low perfusion state is supported by the characteristic 'muddy' granular casts seen on urinary sediment examination (**76**), and the high urinary sodium and FE_{Na}. However, the timing is wrong. ATN should develop immediately after the ischaemic insult. The aetiology of this patient's ARF is best explained by an intrinsic renal mechanism, aminoglycoside nephrotoxicity.

Aminoglycoside nephrotoxicity is usually associated with non-oliguric ARF with declines in GFR occurring after 7–10 days of treatment with these antibiotics. Aminoglycosides cause tubular cell necrosis primarily in the proximal straight and proximal convoluted tubules. The pathogenesis of ATN due to aminoglycosides is related to their deleterious effects on the composition and transport functions of the proximal tubular cells.

ii. In this case, a 'normal' dose of gentamicin was inappropriately high due to the patient's age. Volume depletion should be rapidly corrected and volume status monitored closely during aminoglycoside administration. Aminoglycoside dose should be based on estimates of renal function which account for the patient's age, weight and gender. Serum aminoglycoside levels should be monitored frequently and dosage adjusted to maintain the desired peak and trough levels. Frequent monitoring of renal function during aminoglycoside therapy is warranted. If bacterial sensitivities permit, less nephrotoxic drugs should be used.

77 i. This man has a neurogenic bladder secondary to spina bifida. In such cases renal failure is usually due to reflux and chronic urinary infection. Less commonly patients may develop secondary amyloidosis.

ii. Many patients with spina bifida will have an ilial conduit, which makes peritoneal dialysis less likely to be successful because of an increased risk of peritonitis and intra-abdominal adhesions. In patients with a ventriculoperitoneal shunt (hydrocephalus) peritonitis could cause meningitis, so CAPD is generally contraindicated.

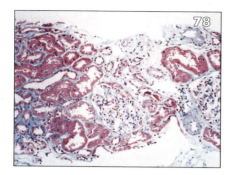

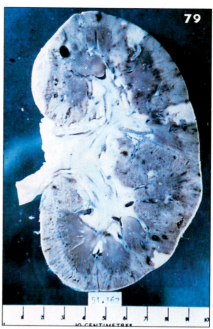

78 A 47-year-old man with ADPKD, who two years previously had undergone a successful renal transplant, presents with a 1-month history of decreasing appetite, increasing fatigue, ankle oedema and nocturia. Following several visits to the transplant clinic, the patient had been lost to follow-up. Physical examination reveals a pale white man with pitting calf oedema. Serum creatinine was 5.7 mg/dl (500 µmol/l), trough cyclosporin A level 200 ng/ml (whole blood HPLC), serum potassium 5.4 mmol/l, and bicarbonate 14 mmol/l. Urinalysis gave a specific gravity of 1.010 and sediment microscopy was unremarkable. A transplant renal biopsy is performed (78).
i. What does the renal biopsy show?
ii. What is the cause of this lesion?
iii. What treatment should be instituted?

79 This nephrectomy specimen (79, courtesy of Dr A. Morley) comes from a 34-year-old woman who developed acute renal failure at 37 weeks of pregnancy. What is the cause of the renal failure?

80 This (80) is the urine sediment light microscopy from a patient with chronic renal failure.
i. What is this abnormality?
ii. What implication does this finding have with respect to the cause of the patient's renal impairment?

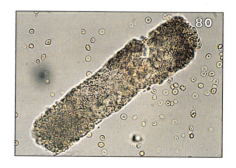

78 i. The biopsy illustrates classic findings of chronic cyclosporin toxicity, i.e., 'striped fibrosis' (areas of relatively normal renal tissue alternating with areas of fibrosis).

ii. The aetiology of chronic cyclosporin nephrotoxicity does not appear to be the result of direct tubular toxicity. Cyclosporin has a direct vasoconstrictor effect on the afferent (pre-glomerular) arteriole, increasing renal vascular resistance and decreasing glomerular filtration rate. The mechanism of afferent arteriolar vasoconstriction is poorly understood, but may be due to decreased synthesis of prostaglandin, a renal vasodilator, or increased production of thromboxane, a vasoconstrictor. Another vasoconstrictor, endothelin, has also been implicated.

The lesions of tubular atrophy and interstitial fibrosis are more likely to occur when the transplanted kidney has been exposed to high trough levels of cyclosporin in the first 6 months following transplant. A direct toxic effect of cyclosporin is supported by the observation of progressive renal insufficiency and similar renal morphological findings in patients without kidney disease who have received cyclosporin therapy for the treatment of uveitis or as immunosuppression following cardiac or liver transplantation.

iii. Generally, renal function will improve if the cyclosporin dose is decreased. The improvement tends to be transient, however, and many of these patients continue to gradually lose renal function, eventually requiring dialysis or retransplantation.

79 There are several wedge-shaped cortical infarcts, typical of cortical necrosis. The most likely underlying cause at this stage of pregnancy is abruptio placenta.

80 i. This is a granular cast.

ii. The finding of granular casts in the urine of a patient with chronic renal failure suggests renal parenchymal disease. Unfortunately, granular casts do not indicate the type of renal pathology. A granular cast is formed when the cells within casts degenerate. This example clearly shows cellular elements within the granularity of the cast. Coarse granularity is probably seen in the early stages of disintegration of the cells, whereas fine granulation implies a longer period within the renal tubule.

81 This 39-year-old woman was treated for 10 years with home haemodialysis.
i. Explain the abnormality (81) noted on inspection of her eyes?
ii. What is the pathogenesis of this complication?
iii. What treatment options are available?

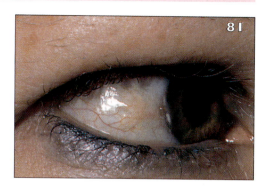

82 An 18-year-old man is found to have a blood pressure of 190/116 mmHg at a routine medical examination. On examination he is found to have a skin rash (82).
i. What is the skin rash?
ii. Is there any possible relationship between this and the raised blood pressure?
iii. What investigations would you undertake in this patient?

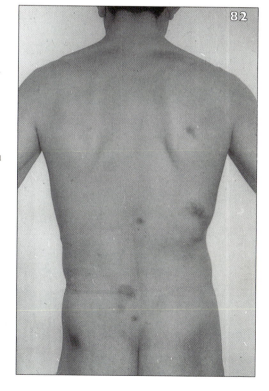

81 i. This long-term haemodialysis patient has corneal calcification. Soft tissue calcification is common in patients with end-stage renal failure. Calcification may involve the sclera (band keratopathy), conjunctiva, joints (chondrocalcinosis), skin, lungs and heart. Such calcification is usually asymptomatic, but may result in conjunctival irritation ('pink eyes'), pruritus, arthralgia, cardiac conduction defects, congestive cardiac failure and pulmonary perfusion–ventilation abnormalities. Visceral calcification is composed of amorphous microcrystals of calcium, phosphate and magnesium. Tumoral and vascular calcification in patients with end-stage renal failure is discussed in **64**.

ii. Soft tissue calcifications are most likely caused by prolonged elevation of the blood calcium/phosphate product. Severe secondary or tertiary hyperparathyroidism, hypermagnesaemia, alkalosis and local tissue injury all predispose the patient to soft tissue calcification.

iii. Meticulous control of plasma phosphate concentration (with appropriate dietary restrictions, the use of oral phosphate binders and adequate haemodialysis prescription and delivery) is preventative. However, phosphate control often proves difficult and in many patients the response to treatment of established soft tissue calcification is disappointing. Phosphate control and medical treatment of secondary hyperparathyroidism are essential. However, symptomatic improvement may take many months despite satisfactory biochemical results. Parathyroidectomy may be necessary to control hyperparathryroidism, or to treat hyperphosphataemia which is refractory to other measures. Mobilisation of soft tissue calcification tends to be less successful in tumoral and vascular distribution (see **64**).

82 i. Visible are café au lait spots and neurofibromata characteristic of neurofibromatosis.

ii. Neurofibromatosis is associated with renal artery stenosis and phaeochromocytoma.

iii. Phaeochromocytoma should be excluded by analysing three 24-hour urine collections for catecholamines. If these are normal, then renal artery stenosis should be excluded. Renal angiography is still the 'gold standard' in cases where there is a high index of suspicion.

83 i. What is this blind diabetic patient doing (83)?

ii. What are the advantages of peritoneal compared with haemodialysis for the uraemic diabetic?

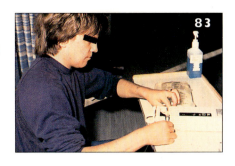

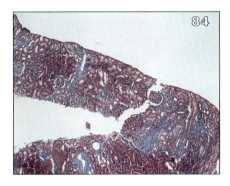

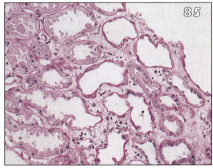

84 Four years after receiving a mismatched renal transplant from her husband, a patient develops a gradual rise in serum creatinine associated with a urinary protein excretion of 560 mg/day. Her maintenance immunosuppressive regimen included prednisone 7.5 mg/day and CSA 5.1 mg/kg/day. A renal biopsy was performed (84).

i. What does the biopsy show?

ii. What treatment would be appropriate?

85 A 72-year-old women with a 10-year history of NIDDM has increasing problems with intermittent claudication. An aortogram is performed. During the next 4 days oliguria is noted and the serum creatinine increases from 1.9 mg/dl (165 µmol/l) to 4.7 mg/dl (420 µmol/l). A renal biopsy is obtained (85). What does the renal biopsy show and what is the underlying problem?

83 i. This patient is using an ultraviolet box to sterilise connections during exchanges. This and the sterile weld device were developed to prevent peritonitis in high-risk patients. They have been largely superseded by the disconnect systems, which have been shown to reduce the incidence of peritonitis.

ii. Creation of conventional vascular access for haemodialysis may be difficult in diabetic patients because of peripheral vascular disease. Insulin may be given intraperitoneally rather than subcutaneously in patients treated by peritoneal dialysis, although improved diabetic control by this route is unproved. Avoidance of anticoagulation during haemodialysis by using peritoneal dialysis might reduce the incidence of retinal and vitreous haemorrhage, although avoidance of hypertension and regular ophthalmological review are more important factors. Metabolic and blood pressure fluctuations should be less in patients who receive continuous peritoneal rather than intermittent haemodialysis. Despite these potential advantages, improved survival and reduced morbidity have not been demonstrated when comparing CAPD with haemodialysis in diabetic patients; indeed, recent analyses suggest that there may be improved outcome with haemodialysis.

84 i. The biopsy demonstrates the 'striped fibrosis' characteristic of long-term CSA nephrotoxicity. It is thought to be secondary to ischaemia resulting from chronic vasoconstriction induced by chronic stimulation of vasoactive substances like endothelin and other inflammatory mediators. In addition, the production of profibrogenic cytokines, including TGF-beta, are also stimulated by CSA and have been implicated in the pathogenisis of interstitial fibrosis. Typically, the vascular lesions are seen only in the smaller renal vessels, e.g., arteriole. Thus, a vasculopathy involving interlobular or arcuate arteries, as seen with chronic rejection or hypertensive nephrosclerosis, can be distinguished from that of chronic CSA or FK506-induced nephrotoxicity.

ii. Downwards adjustment of CSA dosage is usually appropriate, although it is important to maintain adequate immunosuppression, with whole blood CSA levels typically in the range 150–250 ng/ml. The use of a calcium channel blocker may provide some benefit, by reducing CSA-induced afferent arteriolar vasoconstriction and ischaemia, although the evidence remains inconclusive. While the long-term use of CSA can cause irreversible renal injury, it is important to recognise that many more renal allografts are lost to chronic rejection and inadequate immunosuppression than to CSA-induced nephrotoxicity.

85 The renal biopsy shows changes typical of ATN, of which intravenous contrast media is a common cause. The risk factors for this include old age, pre-existing renal disease and diabetes. Unlike atheroembolic disease, in which it may take several weeks before renal failure develops, ATN secondary to intravenous contrast occurs immediately following the radiological procedure. The prognosis is good except for those patients with severe underlying chronic renal disease and diabetes.

86 A patient presents to the emergency room with a fever of 40°C, blood pressure 80/60 mmHg, and heart rate 130 b.p.m. The patient states he has been home vomiting for several days. His WBC is 27,000 x 10^9/l with a marked shift to the left. Lab results are as follows: Na^+ 140 mmol/l, K^+ 3.1 mmol/l, HCO_3^- 24 mEq/l, Cl^- 89 mmol/l, creatinine 1.4 mg/dl (124 µmol/l) and BUN 21 mg/dl (7.5 mmol/l), pH 7.50 and arterial blood gases were pCO_2 27 mmHg, pO_2 81 mmHg. Which best describes the patient's acid–base status?
i. Pure respiratory alkalosis.
ii. Respiratory alkalosis with metabolic acidosis.
iii. Respiratory alkalosis, metabolic acidosis, metabolic alkalosis.
iv. Respiratory alkalosis, metabolic alkalosis.

87 Shown here (**87a**) is a young man who presented with asymptomatic microscopic haematuria and proteinuria. He underwent a renal biopsy and the EM is shown (**87b**, courtesy of Dr A Morley).
i. What comments would you make about his facial appearance?
ii. What abnormality is shown on the EM and what is the primary renal disease?

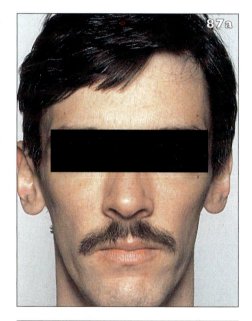

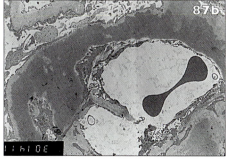

86 iii The patient appears to be in septic shock. When trying to unravel complex acid–base problems, a systematic approach is mandatory. Although no single approach is 'best', all of the following should be evaluated (Table):

- pH – is the patient alkalaemic or acidaemic? If one or the other is present, at least a primary alkalosis or acidosis is present. In this patient, pH is 7.5 and therefore a primary alkalosis is present.
- pCO_2 – if the patient is alkalaemic and the pCO_2 is decreased, a primary respiratory alkalosis is present. If the patient is alkalaemic and the pCO_2 is increased, then a primary metabolic alkalosis is present. In this patient who is alkalaemic with a decrease in his pCO_2 we can conclude that he has a primary respiratory alkalosis.
- HCO_3^- – note that this patient has a normal serum HCO_3^- despite the presence of a respiratory alkalosis. In contrast, we would have expected the serum bicarbonate to decrease to about 18 mmHg to compensate for the respiratory alkalosis [i.e., pCO_2 40 – 27 = 13 x 0.5 mEq/(mmHg pCO_2) = 6.5; 24 – 6.5 = 18.5 mmHg). Thus, given the history of vomiting, a superimposed metabolic alkalosis is likely.
- Anion gap – the last step is to check the anion gap [$(Na^+) – (HCO_3^-) + Cl^-$]. This patient's anion gap is clearly increased (i.e., 27) so, by definition, an anion gap acidosis is present. The most likely scenario is that this patient initially developed a hypochloraemic, hypokalaemic metabolic alkalosis from vomiting and then septic shock, which resulted in an anion gap metabolic and acidosis primary respiratory alkalosis.

Normal compensation	
Metabolic alkalosis	Each 1 mEq increase in HCO_3^- increases pCO_2 ca 0.5–0.8 mmHg
Respiratory alkalosis (chronic)	Each 1 mmHg decrease in pCO_2 decreases HCO_3^- ca 0.5 mEq
Metabolic acidosis	Each 1 mEq decrease in HCO_3^- decreases pCO_2 ca 0.8–1.0 mmHg
Respiratory acidosis (chronic)	Each 1 mmHg increase in pCO_2 increases HCO_3^- ca 0.3–0.6 mEq

87 i. This young man has partial lipodystrophy, which is characterised by loss of subcutaneous tissue from the face, trunk and arms. It is sometimes associated with a viral illness in childhood. Complement abnormalities, including a low C3 and the presence of C3 nephritic factor, are found in some patients and are thought to predispose to the development of mesangiocapillary nephritis.

ii. The EM shows deposits within the basement characteristic of dense deposit disease (Type II mesangiocapillary glomerulonephritis).

88 A 35-year-old man with a history of insulin-dependent diabetes mellitus and mild renal insufficiency [serum creatinine 2.0 mg/dl (175 μmol/l)] presents with left great toe pain of 3 days' duration. On examination the toe is erythematous, swollen and tender. The remainder of the physical examination is unremarkable. Uric acid level is elevated at 10.1 mg/dl (600 μmol/l), but the rest of the laboratory investigations are normal. Joint fluid is obtained and shows uric acid crystals. The patient receives colchicine and ibuprofen. The patient's joint complaints and physical findings resolve, but he returns 7 days later with complaints of 'skipped beats'. An ECG is obtained of which leads V4–6 are shown (**88**, courtesy of Raymond M. Rault). Laboratory values are sodium 136 mmol/l, potassium 6.4 mmol/l, chloride 107 mmol/l, bicarbonate 18 mmol/l, BUN 59 mg/dl (21 mmol/l), urine Na 35 mmol/l, creatinine 2.3 mg/dl (200 μmol/l), urine K^+ 20 mmol/l, uric acid 450 μmol/l (7.6 mg/dl), urine pH 5.0. ABG are pH 7.32, pO_2 99 mmHg, pCO_2 33 mmHg.

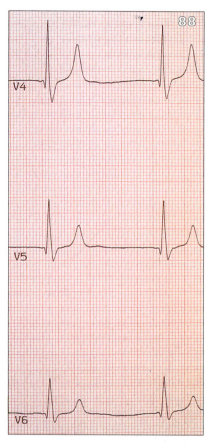

i. What is the aetiology of the patient's hyperkalaemia and elevated serum creatinine?
ii. What is the cause of the patient's acidaemia?

89 A 3-month-old girl presents with a fever of 40°C. The urinalysis reveals numerous white cells and the urine culture grows *E. coli*. The patient is admitted and treated with intravenous antibiotics and her fever resolves in 72 hours. A VCUG is performed (**89**). What does the VCUG demonstrate and what is the appropriate timing for the urological evaluation in this patient?

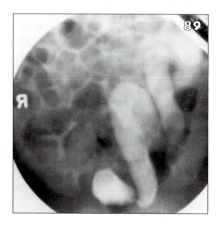

88 i. The use of a NSAID is responsible for the hyperkalaemia and deterioration in renal function. NSAIDs inhibit cyclo-oxygenase activity and decrease prostaglandin production. Prostaglandins have a number of effects on the kidney. They stimulate renin production, thus activating the angiotensin–aldosterone system. Through the action of aldosterone, potassium excretion in the distal tubule is enhanced. In patients with diabetes, as in this case, there is a 30–40% incidence of hyporenin–hypoaldosteronism (Type IV RTA). Inhibition of prostaglandin release by NSAIDs further diminishes renin release, so less angiotensin II is formed, resulting in reduced production of aldosterone. Diminished aldosterone causes decreased potassium secretion by the distal convoluted tubule and collecting duct, resulting in hyperkalaemia. Under normal circumstances prostaglandins have little effect on renal blood flow or GFR. However, when renin production is stimulated (low-salt diet, diuretic use, ischaemia) prostaglandins reduce renal vascular resistance, preserving renal blood flow and preventing renal ischaemic damage. In the face of NSAID-induced prostaglandin inhibition, renal vasoconstriction is unopposed, renal blood flow decreases and renal function deteriorates. This is most likely to occur when maintenance of GFR is dependent upon an activated renin–angiotensin system, such as in individuals with pre-existing renal insufficiency, dehydration, or effective circulating volume depletion due to congestive heart failure, cirrhosis or nephrosis. Rarely, NSAIDs may also cause acute interstitial nephritis, papillary necrosis and the nephrotic syndrome.

The peaked T waves and widening of the QRS complex seen on the ECG are characteristic of hyperkalaemia.

ii. The patient has a non-anion gap metabolic acidosis resulting from decreased hydrogen ion excretion due to the patient's renal insufficiency. Furthermore, this diabetic patient may also have a Type IV RTA. The serum HCO_3^- above 15 mmol/l and the urine pH less than 5.5 support this diagnosis. The inhibition of prostaglandin-mediated renin release by NSAIDs further decreases aldosterone production, decreasing hydrogen ion secretion and exacerbating the acidosis.

89 This is a common presentation for a newborn girl with a urinary tract infection. At the time of initial diagnosis it is appropriate to obtain a renal ultrasound, since this is a non-invasive procedure. In this infant, the ultrasound showed left-sided hydronephrosis. It would also be reasonable to obtain a VCUG, although the exact timing of this procedure remains controversial. In the past, it was recommended to wait until approximately 6 weeks following the urinary tract infection before proceeding with the cystogram. More recently, VCUGs have been performed after the child is afebrile and the repeat urine culture is negative. It would also be important to obtain a a nuclear renogram to assess her renal function and upper urinary tract. In this case, the VCUG revealed a grossly dilated and tortuous left ureter and severe vesicoureteral reflux, which will require surgical reconstruction.

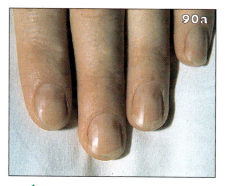
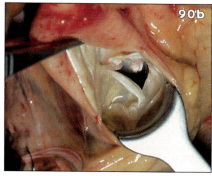

90 This patient (90a, 90b) has had fever for 1 month. What is the diagnosis?

91 A 40-year-old woman presents with excruciating right-flank pain which radiates to her groin. She has a history of recurrent urinary tract infections. At the age of 10 years, she passed a kidney stone and at that time had a normal IVP. A renal ultrasound now reveals bilaterally enlarged cystic kidneys and right-sided hydronephrosis with dilatation of the proximal ureter. An abdominal radiograph shows no obvious kidney stone. Which of the following is she most likely to have?
i. Calcium phosphate stones.
ii. Calcium oxalate stones.
iii. Uric acid stones.
iv. Cysteine stones.
v. Struvite stones.

92 i. What is shown in 92?
ii. What are the treatment options?

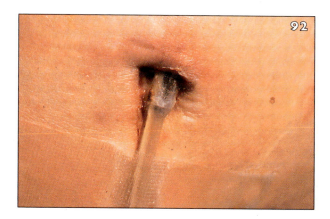

90 Infective endocarditis involving the aortic valve.

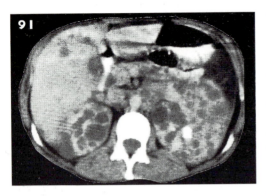

91 iii. Uric acid stones – nephrolithiasis occurs in up to 20% of ADPKD patients. The distorted renal architecture, large cystic structures and calcified cyst walls present in ADPKD mean that radiological documentation of a kidney stone or obstruction is much more difficult. In contrast to the general population, who predominantly form calcium oxalate stones, ADPKD patients develop *uric acid stones* in more than 50% of cases. CT scans may be more sensitive than ultrasonography or IVP for detecting these radiolucent stones (as in **91**, revealing a calculus located in the left collecting system of a patient with ADPKD).

A 24-hour urine metabolic screen usually reveals a low urinary citrate concentration. Citrate complexes with urinary calcium and prevents calcium precipitation. Whether hypocitruria in ADPKD is related to renal tubular acidification defects, as in other autosomally transmitted distal renal tubular acidoses, is not known. Hyperuricosuria and hypercalciuria have also been documented in ADPKD stone formers. All treatment modalities (cystoscopy, percutaneous nephrostomy, extracorporeal shock-wave lithotripsy) are more problematic in ADPKD patients. Complications of such procedures include urinary tract infection from instrumentation, traumatic cyst haemorrhage and obstructing or infected residual stone fragments following lithotripsy.

92 i. The external cuff of this patient's CAPD catheter (which has been partially shaved) is extruding from the subcutaneous tunnel and there is an associated exit-site infection. Cuff extrusion occurs when the external cuff is positioned too near the exit site, when the catheter is inserted with the subcutaneous portion bent out of its natural shape or when the external portion of the catheter is subjected to repeated pulling.
ii. Shaving the cuff off the catheter may be all that is required, as this will prevent further irritation and infection at the exit site. In the presence of exit-site infection, such as illustrated here, shaving the cuff and antibiotic therapy may be ineffective and one should be prepared to replace the catheter.

93 A 55-year-old man with a 15-year history of non-insulin dependent diabetes mellitus (NIDDM) develops proteinuria and renal insufficiency. His medications include an oral hypoglycaemic agent and a calcium-channel blocker. His blood pressure is 140/85 mmHg, he has decreased position and vibratory sensation in his feet, 1+ pitting lower-extremity oedema and evidence of previous retinal photocoagulation. His urinary protein excretion is 900 mg/day. His laboratory values are: serum sodium 142 mmol/l, potassium 5.6 mmol/l, chloride 114 mmol/l, bicarbonate 18 mmol/l, creatinine 2.0 mg/dl (177 μmol/l), urea nitrogen 30 mg/dl (10.7 mmol/l); arterial blood gas pH 7.36, [H^+] 44 nmol/l (38–42 nmol/l), pCO_2 33 mmHg.
i. What is the aetiology of his acid–base disorder?
ii. What therapy would you recommend?

94 This patient had endocarditis (see 90) and has now developed renal impairment with haematuria and proteinuria.
i. The renal biopsy is shown (94) – what is the diagnosis?
ii. What other causes of acute renal failure may there be in association with endocarditis?

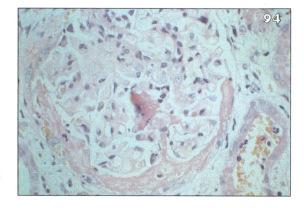

95 A renal transplant recipient presented with fever and melena, and required transfusion with four units of packed red blood cells. Upper gastrointestinal endoscopy was performed, and multiple superficial mucosal ulcerations seen (95).
i. What is the most likely diagnosis in this patient?
ii. What is the differential diagnosis of gastrointestinal bleeding in a renal transplant recipient?

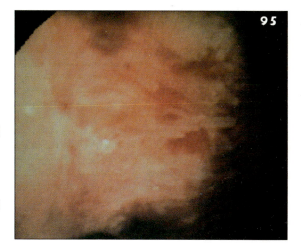

93 i. The patient has hyperkalaemia and a normal anion-gap metabolic acidosis. The most likely aetiology is type IV RTA secondary to diabetic nephropathy. Type IV RTA results from impaired acid secretion secondary to aldosterone deficiency or resistance. Hyperkalaemia develops due to impaired potassium secretion by the cortical collecting tubule due to a lack of aldosterone effect. Without aldosterone the lumen is less electronegative and a favourable gradient does not exist for secretion of potassium or H^+ ions. Hyperkalaemia exacerbates the metabolic acidosis by inhibiting renal ammonia genesis, further decreasing hydrogen ion excretion. Other disorders that can cause Type IV RTA include aldosterone deficiency due to Addison's disease or heparin therapy, medications (spironolactone, triamterene, amiloride, lithium) and chronic interstitial nephritis (e.g., analgesics, allergy, sarcoid, lupus, etc.).
ii. Therapy for Type IV RTA includes a low-potassium diet and the use of loop diuretics to increase distal sodium delivery favouring potassium and H^+ excretion. Oral sodium bicarbonate can also be used to correct the metabolic acidosis and to increase distal sodium delivery.

94 i. The patient has focal segmental necrotising glomerulonephritis *consistent* with infective endocarditis – often called 'SBE nephritis' (subacute bacterial endocarditis). However, the renal biopsy is not diagnostic as similar patterns may be seen in other disorders, particularly systemic vasculitis. In endocarditis, glomerular deposits of C3 and low serum C3 are characteristic, but not universal, and may be accompanied by IgG and IgM; in systemic vasculitis the glomerular histology typically reveals minimal or no glomerular deposits (i.e., pauci-immune). The therapeutic approach in vasculitis – intense immunosuppression – is absolutely contraindicated in endocarditis, so in equivocal cases endocarditis must be assiduously excluded by echocardiography and repeated blood cultures.
ii. ATN may follow renal hypoperfusion due to impaired cardiac function. Gentamicin nephrotoxicity may occur, particularly if this antibiotic is combined with loop diuretics. Occasionally, cardiac vegetations embolise to the kidney causing micro- or macro-infarcts. Typically, there is other clinical evidence of emboli (cerebrovascular accident, peripheral cutaneous infarcts, haematuria, flank pain).

95 i. Gastrointestinal bleeding is common in renal transplant recipients. This patient had CMV gastroenteritis. CMV can cause mucosal damage virtually anywhere in the gastrointestinal tract, i.e., in the oesophagus, stomach, duodenum, jejunum and colon.
ii. In addition to CMV enteritis, oesophagitis, gastritis, gastric and duodenal ulcers, and colonic neoplasms are common causes of gastrointestinal bleeding in transplant recipients.

96 i. What does this renal angiogram (**96**) show?
ii. What are the causes of this condition?
iii. How would you confirm the diagnosis?

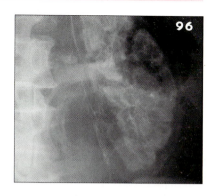

97 Shown (**97**) is the CT scan of a 55-year-old man who presented with malaise, backache and advanced uraemia. An ultrasound performed on admission showed bilateral hydronephrosis.
i. What does the CT scan show?
ii. What could be the aetiology of this abnormality?

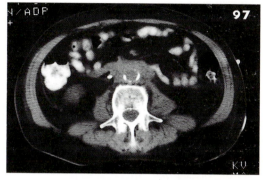

98 This 3-year-old boy has 4+ protein in his urine on stick testing. His serum albumin is 21 g/l.
i. What is the most likely diagnosis?
ii. This photograph (**98**) was taken at 9.00, but by lunchtime his facial oedema had resolved – why?

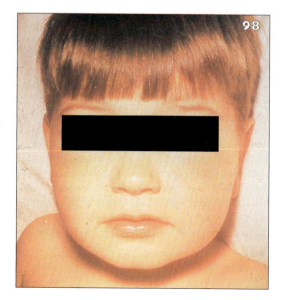

96 i. The angiogram shows cortical necrosis with no perfusion of the cortex other than a capsular rim. This patient had bilateral renal cortical necrosis and irreversible renal failure.

ii. Obstetric complications are the most common cause of bilateral renal cortical necrosis (BRCN), which may occur in early pregnancy after septic abortion or, more commonly, in late pregnancy after placental abruption. It is suggested clinically by prolonged severe oliguria lasting 20 days or more. Obstetric causes of ARF have become increasingly rare in developed countries over recent decades: statistics from Dublin showed an incidence of BRCN of 1 in 80,000 deliveries between 1971 and 1980, compared with 1 in 10,000 deliveries between 1961 and 1970. BRCN remains more common in underdeveloped countries – a recent series from India described 23 cases of BRCN from 1985–1992; 15 were due to obstetric causes.

iii. Renal biopsy will demonstrate necrotic glomeruli. Patchy cortical necrosis, which has a better prognosis, may be missed on renal biopsy, so arteriography or a CT scan may be required to demonstrate it. After 4–6 weeks, cortical calcification may be seen on plain abdominal radiography.

97 i. The CT scan shows a retroperitoneal mass.

ii. Possible causes of this include idiopathic or drug-induced (methysergide) retroperitoneal fibrosis, an abdominal aortic aneurysm and retroperitoneal lymphoma. In this case biopsy showed retroperitoneal fibrosis, which is more common in men. It often presents insidiously with general malaise, backache, anaemia and uraemia. Dense retroperitoneal tissue causes obstruction of one or both kidneys. The earliest sign on IVP is medial deviation of one or both ureters, progressing to ureteric obstruction, usually at the junction between the middle and lower third of the ureter. Treatment includes either corticosteroids or ureteral diversion.

98 i. This boy has nephrotic syndrome. The most common cause in a child of this age is minimal change nephrotic syndrome, in which case the proteinuria will usually resolve completely with corticosteroid therapy. Another diagnosis should be suspected if there is microscopic haematuria, hypertension or renal impairment at presentation. However, these are not absolute criteria – about 10% of children with minimal change nephrotic syndrome have haematuria, and renal impairment may be present because of volume contraction rather than intrinsic glomerular disease.

ii. Resolution occurs because of the effect of gravity, on which oedema is dependent regardless of the underlying cause. In adults the common cause of widespread oedema is congestive heart failure, in which orthopnoea prevents the patient from sleeping supine and thus restricts oedema to the lower body. The nephrotic child usually has no respiratory limitation to prevent sleeping flat, thus producing facial oedema in the morning.

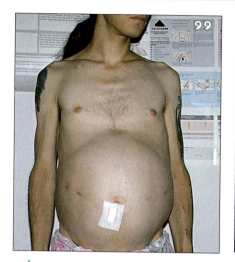

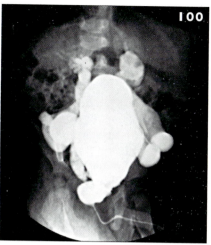

99 This 21-year-old man developed progressive abdominal distension (99) within 1 year of commencing chronic haemodialysis. There was no history or clinical evidence of cardiac, respiratory or hepatic disease.
i. Which dialysis-related complication does this young man demonstrate?
ii. Explain the pathogenesis of this complication?
iii. What treatment options are available?

100 A prenatal ultrasound of a 26-week-old male foetus shows bilateral hydronephrosis and a very enlarged bladder. A VCUG is performed after delivery (100). On examination the abdominal wall appears thin.
i. What is the prenatal differential diagnosis?
ii. What does the VCUG show?
iii. What is the underlying diagnosis?

101 This 34-year-old male renal transplant recipient had noted these skin lesions (101) for the past several years and states that they developed shortly after receiving his kidney transplant.
i. What are these lesions?
ii. What complications can be associated?

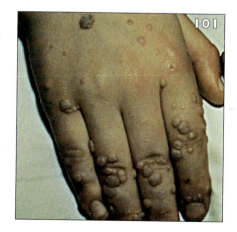

99 i. This man has dialysis ascites, defined as the development of ascites without discernible cause in a patient maintained on chronic haemodialysis treatment. This diagnosis is established by the exclusion of other causes of ascites (e.g., congestive cardiac failure, constrictive pericarditis, liver cirrhosis, abdominal malignancies, tuberculous peritonitis, etc.) by careful clinical examination, cardiac ultrasound, CT, laparoscopy and even laparotomy. Ascitic fluid should be examined for protein concentration, amylase concentration, cytology and cell count, as well as culture for bacterial, fungal and mycobacterial organisms. Ascitic fluid in dialysis ascites is typically exudative and straw yellow in colour.

ii. The pathogenesis of dialysis ascites is unknown. Serositis due to advanced uraemia or chronic hyperparathyroidism, previous damage to the peritoneum during peritoneal dialysis, overhydration and hypoalbuminaemia may all be contributory.

iii. Haemodialysis-related ascites should be treated aggressively. The first approach to treatment is aggressive fluid management, with sodium and water restriction, and intensive haemodialysis and ultrafiltration. Hypotension, unfortunately, is a frequent limiting factor. On occasion, laparotomy, performed as part of the investigative process, is followed by remission of the ascites. The best therapeutic response, however, is achieved either by a transfer of the patient to peritoneal dialysis or by renal transplantation.

100 i. The differential diagnosis of hydronephrosis in a male foetus includes posterior urethral valves, prune-belly syndrome, urethral atresia and vesicoureteral reflux. However, with the information provided these possibilities cannot be differentiated. If the amount of amniotic fluid is normal by ultrasonography, the patient can be followed expectantly.

ii. The VCUG shows a grossly enlarged bladder, tortuous dilated ureters and bilateral hydronephrosis.

iii. This is a classic picture for the prune-belly syndrome. It is important that *in utero* intervention *not* be attempted in these patients, since the degree of hydronephrosis may not accurately reflect the loss of renal function.

101 i. Common warts are present in nearly half of renal transplant recipients and are secondary to the reactivation of latent human papillomaviruses (HPV) in response to immunosuppressive therapy. While immunosuppressive therapy is continued, eradication is unusual. Measures to control these lesions include periodic surgical or chemical debridement and avoidance of other non-specific irritants, such as excessive ultraviolet light exposure.

ii. Squamous cell carcinomas of the skin have been found to contain viral material from certain types of HPV, such as HPV Type 5, and a causal linkage has been postulated. HPV has also been associated with cervical carcinoma, a malignancy whose incidence in the transplant population is 15-fold greater than that in the general population. Careful monitoring for malignant transformations is therefore appropriate for all transplant patients known to be infected with these organisms.

102 A 31-year-old woman presents with a 1-month history of headaches, increased thirst and urinary frequency. Urine output over 24 hours was 8 litres. The patient was admitted to the hospital and, under careful observation, a brief fluid deprivation test was performed (see Table).

i. Which is the most likely diagnosis: psychogenic polydipsia, nephrogenic diabetes insipidus, central diabetes insipidus or surreptitious diuretic use?

ii. Which of the following treatments may be of benefit?

(a) Hydrochlorothiazide.

(b) Desmopressin.

(c) Frusemide (furosemide).

Time	Serum Na$^+$ (mmol/l)	Urine osmolarity (mOsm/l)	Serum ADH (pg/ml)	Urine output (ml)
Baseline	144	80	2	–
I hour	147	80	2	600
2 hour	150	80	2	500
Test ended				

103 A 49-year-old patient with end-stage renal failure experienced profound hypotension during a regular haemodialysis session, despite peripheral oedema and being 2 kg above his 'dry weight'. Clinical examination revealed mild pyrexia, elevated jugular venous pressure and a paradoxical pulse.

i. What abnormality does the patient's chest radiograph (103) show?

ii. What treatment options are available?

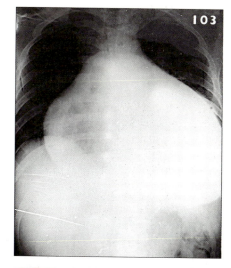

104 i. What is shown in **104**?

ii. How is this investigation used?

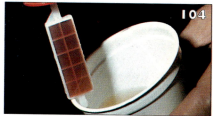

102 i. This patient has central diabetes insipidus and her defect appears to be quite severe. The differential diagnosis should include both central and nephrogenic diabetes insipidus, as well as psychogenic polydipsia and diuretic use. In all of these cases, maximal urinary concentrating ability may be impaired, although severe impairment, as in this case, is suggestive of central diabetes insipidus. In diagnosing these disorders, either a fluid deprivation test or hypertonic saline challenge should be performed. In both instances, the goal is to increase serum osmolarity sufficiently to stimulate ADH secretion. In psychogenic polydipsia and diuretic use, urine osmolarity should rise significantly, although it may not increase to normal secondary to medullary washout. In both central and nephrogenic diabetes insipidus, the urine osmolarity may not rise. The discriminant point is that in response to the fluid deprivation test ADH levels remain low in central diabetes insipidus ,but increase in nephrogenic diabetes insipidus. Alternatively, desmopressin could be administered instead of obtaining serum ADH levels. In central diabetes insipidus, urine osmolarity will increase following the administration of desmopressin, whereas in nephrogenic diabetes insipidus, it will not.
ii. (b) In central diabetes insipidus, desmopressin is the preferred treatment. Hydrochlorothiazide, by inducing mild volume depletion and decreasing distal nephron water delivery, can decrease polyuria significantly in nephrogenic diabetes insipidus. Frusemide (furosemide) would not be indicated in the treatment of central diabetes insipidus.

103 i. The radiograph demonstrates gross enlargement of the cardiac silhouette with clear lung fields. The physical signs suggests a pericardial effusion causing cardiac tamponade.
ii. The frequency of pericarditis in haemodialysis patients correlates with plasma urea, creatinine and phosphate concentrations, suggesting that uraemic pericarditis is a marker of inadequate renal replacement therapy. Most patients have an associated pericardial effusion, which may cause cardiac tamponade. Symptoms may be precipitated by reduction of blood volume during ultrafiltration, or from haemopericardium during heparinisation on dialysis. In this situation emergency pericardiocentesis may be life-saving.

Uraemic pericarditis usually responds to intensification of dialysis therapy. Daily haemodialysis with low-dose or no heparin, or a conversion to peritoneal dialysis to avoid anticoagulation, are treatment options.

104 i. Shown is a patient removing a dip slide from a mid-stream urine sample. Dip slides consist of a plastic mount covered on one side with MacConkey's medium and on the other with CLED medium. Patients are instructed to dip the slide into the sample and then forward it to their physician or the microbiology laboratory.
ii. Dip slides are used in the assessment of patients with symptoms suggestive of recurrent urinary infection. They are also useful in assessing the efficacy of antibiotics in recurrent urinary tract infections.

105 A 65-year-old man is brought to the hospital by his family. He has been confined to bed for the past several days due to severe nausea and vomiting and has been unable to take anything by mouth. Despite this he has maintained a good urine output throughout his illness. The patient has manic-depressive illness and has been taking lithium carbonate for 15 years. On physical examination, he is lethargic but able to communicate. Vital signs show a temperature of 37.9°C, a pulse of 125 b.p.m., a respiratory rate of 16 breaths per minute and a supine blood pressure of 100/60 mmHg, which fell to 70/40 mmHg in the sitting position. The remainder of the physical examination is normal. Laboratory studies show plasma lithium 1.5 mmol/l; urea nitrogen, 7.0 mmol/l (20 mg/dl); creatinine level, 130 μmol/l (1.5 mg/dl); serum sodium, 169 mmol/l; serum calcium 2.3 mmol/l; serum glucose 4 mmol/l and urine osmolarity, 240 mOsm/l. Discuss the probable aetiology of the patient's hypernatraemia, polyuria and polydipsia.

106 A 60-year-old woman is referred for progressive renal insufficiency. She has mild anaemia and thrombocytopenia. Serum creatinine is 4 mg/dl (354 μmol/l), serum albumin 31 g/l and total protein 65 g/l. Urinalysis reveals 4+ protein, 20–30 RBCs (20% of them dysmorphic) and 2+ granular casts. Serum and urine protein electrophoresis are shown in **106a**. Serum immunofixation is illustrated in **106b**.
i. How would you interpret those results?
ii. What renal lesions could be associated with these findings?

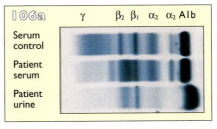

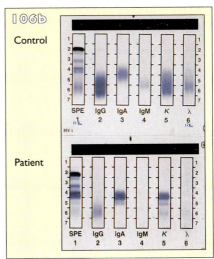

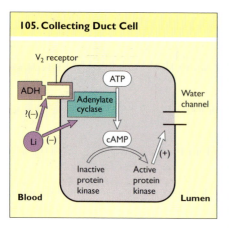

105. Collecting Duct Cell

V_2 receptor

ADH

?(−)

Li (−)

ATP

Adenylate cyclase

cAMP

Inactive protein kinase

Active protein kinase

Water channel

(+)

Blood

Lumen

105 This patient has a defect in renal water reabsorbtion as indicated by the failure to increase urinary osmolality in the face of a marked increase in serum osmolality. The differential diagnosis in this case would be a lack of ADH production (central diabetes insipidus) or a failure of the kidney to respond to ADH (nephrogenic diabetes insipidus). Lithium carbonate therapy is frequently associated with urinary concentrating defects, causing overt nephrogenic diabetes insipidus in 5–20% of patients, increased thirst in 70%, polydipsia in 40%, polyuria in 2–35% and impaired maximal urinary concentrating ability in 30–90%. Nephrogenic diabetes insipidus is thought to result from the interference of lithium carbonate with cAMP generation by ADH's action on adenylate cyclase in the collecting tubule (see **105**). Lithium may also interfere with the action of ADH at its receptor site. Failure of ADH to increase water permeability in the cortical and medullary collecting tubules leads to a urinary concentrating defect. The loss of free water increases serum osmolality, which increases thirst. In this case the patient was able to compensate for the increased urinary losses by increasing his fluid intake until intercurrent illness prevented it.

Other drugs which cause nephrogenic diabetes insipidus include amphotericin B and demeclocycline.

106 i. In **106a**, serum protein electrophoresis demonstrates an abnormal band in the β_1–β_2 region, which could represent a paraprotein. Total immunoglobulins are also decreased. On immunofixation (**106b**), an IgA kappa paraprotein is identified and the concentration of IgG and IgM are reduced. Urine electrophoresis (**106a**, bottom lane) reveals a band in the β_2 region that comigrates with the serum band, as well as significant amounts of albumin, indicative of glomerular proteinuria.

ii. Three renal lesions could be associated with this presentation: (a) myeloma kidney, (b) light chain nephropathy, and (c) primary amyloidosis. A kidney biopsy is necessary to differentiate between the three diagnoses. In myeloma kidney, light chains coprecipitate with Tamm–Horsfall protein and cause distal tubular obstruction. These myeloma casts have a characteristic refractile, 'fractured' appearance on light microscopy. In light chain nephropathy, monoclonal light chains deposit in the glomerulus, mesangium, vessels and tubular cells. Other organs, especially the heart, may also be involved. Primary amyloidosis occurs in 10% of myeloma patients, and usually involves other organs as well. In contrast to myeloma kidney, light chain nephropathy and amyloidosis are associated with prominent glomerular deposits, frequently resulting in nephrotic range proteinuria. Final characterisation will depend on the results of Congo red staining, immunofluorescence and electron microscopic studies.

107 A 32-year-old woman developed accelerated hypertension 6 weeks following living related renal allograft. Multiple agents were used to control her blood pressure with little benefit. When an ACE inhibitor was added to the regimen, the patient experienced an acute decline in renal function. A renal arteriogram (**107**) was obtained.

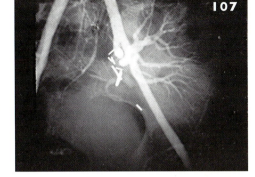

i. What does the arteriogram show?
ii. Would a nuclear renal scan and/or a Doppler ultrasound have been useful as non invasive screening tests?
iii. How should this patient be managed?

108 A 25-year-old man with sickle cell disease (Hgb SS) was admitted with a pain crisis. His blood pressure is 150/70 mmHg, heart rate 115 b.p.m., respirations 28 breaths per minute, and temperature 37°C. He is a thin man with low back tenderness on palpation. The remainder of his examination is normal. He receives narcotic analgesics, intravenous dextrose and water (D5W, 5% dextrose) and bed rest. His laboratory studies on admission and 2 days following resolution of his pain crisis are given (Table).

Serum	Day 1	Day 4
Sodium	140	138
Potassium	4.0	3.8
Chloride	112	108
Total CO_2	16	18

Arterial blood gas	Day 1	Day 4
pH	7.52	7.36
pCO_2	20	33

i. What is the acid–base disturbance on the first day?
ii. What is the acid–base disturbance on the fourth day?
iii. What are the renal complications of sickle-cell disease?

109 Why might this patient (**109**) have developed membranous nephropathy?

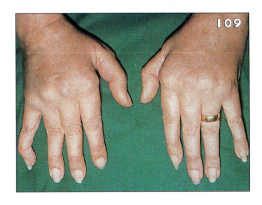

107 i. The arteriogram demonstrates an 80% stenosis with a 50 mmHg gradient at the vascular anastomosis. The potential causes for transplant renal artery stenosis include host factors, such as pre-existing vascular disease, anastomotic technical problems (e.g., clamp injuries or suturing complications) or donor-related complications, such as preservation injury, kinking or angulation, and rejection. In this case, the arteriogram confirmed the clinical suspicion of technical complication at the vascular anastomosis.

ii. A nuclear scan is of limited value in making this diagnosis since there is no contralateral 'control' kidney for comparison. The Doppler ultrasound is limited by variable sensitivity and specificity, which is often operator-dependent. The renal arteriogram remains the 'gold standard'.

iii. Percutaneous transluminal angioplasty is the preferred approach if technically feasible; it can usually be performed at the time of the arteriogram. Success rates are in the range of 80%, although recurrences within 6 months may occur in up to 30% of patients. Surgical revascularisation is usually reserved for technically difficult cases and is associated with an allograft loss rate as high as 30%.

108 i. On the first day he has respiratory alkalosis and metabolic acidosis. The respiratory alkalosis is due to tachypnoea from pain. The presence of metabolic acidosis is suspected because the decrease in serum bicarbonate was greater than would be expected as metabolic compensation for acute respiratory alkalosis. The predicted metabolic compensation for *acute* respiratory alkalosis can be estimated with the equation:

$\Delta HCO_3^- = 0.2 \, (\Delta pCO_2)$

Thus, the predicted change in serum bicarbonate would be:

$\Delta HCO_3^- = 0.2 \, (40 - 20) = 4$

i.e., an expected HCO_3^- of 20 mmol/l rather than the observed 16 mmol/l.

ii. On the fourth day he has a normal anion-gap metabolic acidosis, most likely due to distal (Type I) RTA secondary to sickle cell nephropathy. Evidence for this diagnosis includes: acidaemia (low pH), normal anion gap and appropriate respiratory compensation. Additional evidence that supports distal RTA includes a urine pH >5.5 and a positive urinary anion gap. In sickle-cell anaemia, medullary ischaemia impairs the ability to acidify and concentrate the urine. Other complications of distal RTA include nephrolithiasis and nephrocalcinosis.

iii. Sickle-cell anaemia causes a variety of renal diseases including nephrogenic diabetes insipidus (impaired renal concentrating ability), glomerulonephritis, renal tubular acidosis, haematuria, papillary necrosis and ESRD.

109 The patient has severe rheumatoid arthritis and has probably received disease-modifying ('second-line') drugs. Treatment with gold or penicillamine may induce membranous nephropathy. The natural history is slow regression of proteinuria once the drug is withdrawn, although complete resolution may take more than 10 years.

also NSAIDs.

110 A 36-year-old woman with ADPKD and an asymptomatic cerebral aneurysm presents with moderate hypertension. The preferred antihypertensive drug regimen would include which of the following?
i. Beta-blocker.
ii. Calcium channel blocker.
iii. Diuretic.
iv. ACEI.
v. Alpha-blocker.
vi. Centrally acting sympatholytic agent.

111 A 35-year-old white man is referred to the renal clinic for evaluation of proteinuria. He has no complaints other than swelling at the end of the day and foamy urine. He denies a history of kidney, heart or liver disease. Physical examination is remarkable for a thin man who appears older than his stated age. There are numerous healed 'track marks' over both forearms, but he states that he has not used intravenous drugs for 5 years. He has 3+ pitting oedema of his lower extremities. Urinalysis shows 4+ protein, oval fat bodies and granular casts. His serum creatinine is 6.8 mg/dl (600 μmol/l) and 24-hour urine protein excretion is 5.5 g/day. The patient has normal-sized kidneys by ultrasound and undergoes renal biopsy. Two representative fields are shown in **111a** and **111b** (both stained with methenamine silver trichrome; courtesy Sheldon I. Bastacky). What is the most likely aetiology of the patient's renal disease?

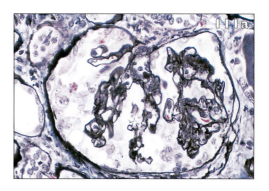

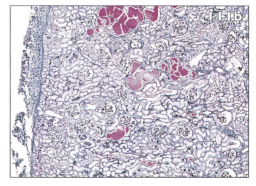

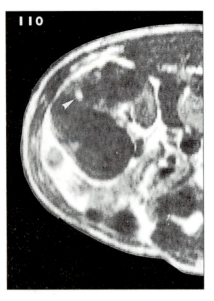

110 iv. ACEI – 60–75% of ADPKD patients with cerebral aneurysms will experience rupture, usually occurring after 50 years of age in individuals with poorly controlled hypertension. Hypertension occurs in 50–70% of patients with ADPKD, often preceding the development of renal insufficiency. Cyst enlargement leading to the compression of intrarenal vasculature (as demonstrated by the MRI, 110) is believed to cause local renal ischaemia, resulting in hyperrenin hyperaldosteronism and secondary hypertension. In addition, the epithelial lining of the cysts has been shown to elaborate renin, which could theoretically lead to angiotensin II-mediated epithelial cell proliferation and hypertrophy.

Consequently, ACEIs are particularly effective for treating hypertension in ADPKD. Haemodynamically mediated ARF is occasionally observed (<5% of cases), but is usually mild and reversible after discontinuing the ACEI. Concomitant diuretic use or cyst haemorrhage may predispose ADPKD patients to this haemodynamically mediated reduction in GFR.

111 111a and 111b demonstrate several of the typical findings of HIV-associated nephropathy. In 111a the glomerular capillaries are globally collapsed and the epithelial cells enlarged and vacuolated. The lower power view in 111b shows microcystic dilatation of renal tubules with pale-staining cast material. On electron microscopy tubuloreticular structures in the glomerular endothelial cells were found. The majority of patients with HIV-associated nephropathy have a variant of focal segmental glomerulosclerosis with the characteristic changes described above.

HIV-associated nephropathy was first described in young black men who abused intravenous drugs. Originally, this condition was thought to be a late manifestation of HIV infection, but it has now been seen at all stages of the infection and in all populations at risk for HIV.

Oedema, hypercholesterolaemia and hypertension are uncommon. The kidneys are usually normal or increased in size on ultrasound. The course to ESRD tends to be rapid in adults. No therapy has proved effective for treatment of HIV nephropathy and life expectancy on dialysis is poor with AIDS patients succumbing within a period of weeks or months. Longer survival has been reported in those patients with asymptomatic HIV infection or AIDS-related complex.

112 A 46-year-old renal allograft recipient sustained a myocardial infarction 3 years after transplantation. His serum creatinine was 1.2 mg/dl (110 µmol/l), and he was taking CSA, prednisone, azathioprine, frusemide (furosemide) and metoprolol.
i. Is the lipid profile shown (Table) unusual for a renal transplant recipient?
ii. What might be contributing to the hyperlipidaemia in this patient?
iii. How would you treat this patient's lipid abnormalities?

Test	Result	Low risk
Total cholesterol	295 mg/dl (7.6 mmol/l)	<200 mg/dl (<5.2 mmol/l)
LDL cholesterol	198 mg/dl (5.1 mmol/l)	<130 mg/dl (<3.4 mmol/l)
HDL cholesterol	55 mg/dl (1.4 mmol/l)	>35 mg/dl (>0.9 mmol/l)
Triglycerides	210 mg/dl (2.4 mmol/l)	<200 mg/dl (<2.3 mmol/l)

113 This (**113**) is the IVP of a 27-year-old woman who was found to be hypertensive during her first pregnancy, necessitating antihypertensive treatment and early delivery of the baby. Serum creatinine was normal.
i. What abnormalities are seen?
ii. What advice would you give about the risk of complications in future pregnancies?

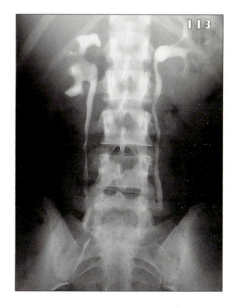

114 A patient underwent renal biopsy one month following a mismatched cadaveric renal transplant because his serum creatinine abruptly rose. His immunosuppressive regimen included prednisone and tacrolimus (FK506).
i. What does the renal biopsy (**114**) show?
ii. How should this patient be treated?

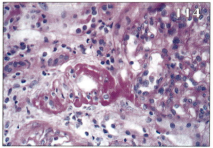

112 i. Hyperlipidaemia is common following renal transplantation. Although increases in LDL cholesterol are especially common, serum triglycerides may be elevated as well. HDL cholesterol levels are usually normal, but are sometimes decreased.
ii. Both corticosteroids and cyclosporin (CSA) have been shown to increase plasma lipid levels. Diuretics and beta-blockers may also play a role. Other clinical correlates include renal dysfunction or allograft rejection, proteinuria, gender and pre-transplant lipid levels.
iii. Increases in LDL cholesterol should probably be treated in patients with multiple cardiovascular risk factors or evidence of atherosclerotic cardiovascular disease. Dietary modification should be used in conjunction with a 3-hydroxy-3-methylglutaryl coenzyme A (HMG-CoA) reductase inhibitor. Initial reports of an increased incidence of myositis and hepatitis in transplant recipients receiving conventional doses of HMG-CoA reductase inhibitors likely reflect increased blood levels due to CSA-induced inhibition of hepatic metabolism. More recent evidence indicates that low doses of HMG-CoA reductase inhibitors can be used safely in transplant recipients receiving CSA.

113 i. The right kidney is small (7 cm) with clubbing of the upper and lower pole calyces with adjacent cortical atrophy. The left kidney appears normal. The changes are those of chronic pyelonephritis (reflux nephropathy).
ii. Reflux nephropathy is one of the most common renal problems in women of child-bearing age; it may be associated with urinary tract infection, hypertension and chronic renal impairment. It can be asymptomatic and may present for the first time during pregnancy. Pregnancy is likely to be uncomplicated if renal function and blood pressure are normal at conception. Careful antenatal screening and prompt treatment of bacteriuria should reduce symptomatic urinary tract infections, which are a frequent cause of maternal morbidity, but a rare cause of foetal mortality. The level of renal function and blood pressure are more important determinants of foetal outcome. Current evidence suggests that if the serum creatinine is less than 200 µmol/l, most pregnancies will be successful. If renal function is worse than this, especially with coexisting hypertension, there is an increased incidence of foetal growth retardation and intrauterine death. There is also a risk of an increased rate of decline of maternal renal function.

114 i. Tacrolimus and cyclosporin can cause similar renal lesions, given their similar mode of action. The biopsy shows arteriolar injury which may be seen with either drug, especially at high doses. The pathophysiology involves myointimal injury with insudation of proteinaceous material.
ii. This lesion is typically found when blood levels of FK506 or cyclosporin are high and is usually managed by carefully decreasing the dosage. In rare instances, more diffuse injury may occur, resulting in thrombotic microangiopathy. In these cases, cessation of the drug or conversion to an alternative immunosuppressive regimen may be necessary.

115 A 60-year-old obese white woman presents with complaints of polyuria and polydipsia for the past several months. She has no other complaints and is on no medication. Her phys-ical examination is unremarkable. The only laboratory abnormalities are a fasting serum glucose of 270 mg/dl (15 mmol/l) and urinalysis revealing 2+ glucose and 1+ protein by dipstick. A fat- and calorie-restricted diet is prescribed and the patient instructed to return in several weeks. Upon return, her symptoms and serum glucose have not improved. Therapy is instituted with chlorpropamide 100 mg once a day.

After 6 weeks the patient returns with complaints of fatigue and nausea. The patient is euvolaemic on examination, with a blood pressure of 130/90 mmHg without orthostatic changes. Her laboratory tests show serum sodium 120 mmol/l, serum uric acid 2.5 mg/dl (150 µmol/l), serum glucose 270 mg/dl (15 mmol/l) and urine osmolality 600 mOsm/l.

i. Comment on the urine osmolarity and serum sodium.
ii. Why is this patient hyponatraemic?

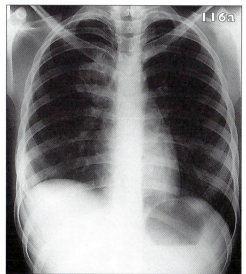

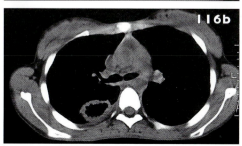

116 A teenage Caucasian girl was referred to a pulmonary specialist with a complaint of general malaise, weight loss, fever and cough. She was also complaining of a painful nose.

i. What do the chest radiograph (**116a**) and thoracic CT scan (**116b**) show?
ii. What is visible on her face (**116c**) and what is the diagnosis?

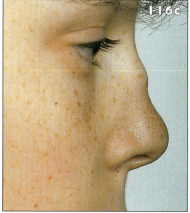

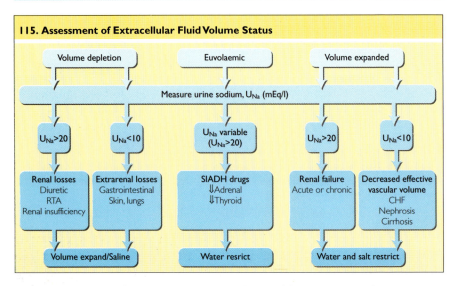

115. Assessment of Extracellular Fluid Volume Status

Volume depletion	Euvolaemic	Volume expanded

Measure urine sodium, U_{Na} (mEq/l)

$U_{Na}>20$	$U_{Na}<10$	U_{Na} variable ($U_{Na}>20$)	$U_{Na}>20$	$U_{Na}<10$
Renal losses Diuretic RTA Renal insufficiency	**Extrarenal losses** Gastrointestinal Skin, lungs	**SIADH drugs** ⇓Adrenal ⇓Thyroid	**Renal failure** Acute or chronic	**Decreased effective vascular volume** CHF Nephrosis Cirrhosis
Volume expand/Saline		**Water resrict**	**Water and salt restrict**	

115 i. The patient is hyponatraemic and has a concentrated urine. In the presence of hyponatraemia (hypo-osmolarity) the urine should be maximally dilute in order to excrete the excess free water.

ii. Illustrated here (**115**) is a diagnostic approach to hyponatraemic disorders. This patient is euvolaemic, narrowing the diagnostic possibilities to glucocorticoid deficiency, hypothyroidism or the syndrome of inappropriate ADH (SIADH). Given the acuity of the decrease in serum sodium, cortisol- or thyroid-deficiency are unlikely. Drug-induced SIADH can occur due to potentiation of the ADH effect (chlorpropamide, carbamezipine, intravenous cyclophosphamide, tolbutamide, NSAIDs) or increased production of ADH (e.g., intravenous cyclophosphamide, vincristine, haloperidol, amitriptyline, thiothixene, narcotics and thioridazine). In this patient chlorpropamide is the most likely cause of drug-induced SIADH. Chlorpropamide-induced hyponatraemia is most likely to occur in diabetics over the age of 60 who are also taking a thiazide diuretic. Studies in animals treated with chlorpropamide show enhanced sodium reabsorption in the medullary ascending limb, which increases medullary tonicity and hence the osmotic driving force for water reabsorption.

116 i. The chest radiograph (**116a**) and thoracic CT scan (**116b**) show a cavitating lesion in the right upper quadrant.

ii. **116c** shows that a 'saddle-nose' deformity. The diagnosis is Wegener's granulomatosis, which is characterised by a necrotising granulomatous inflammation of the upper and lower respiratory tract often associated with a glomerulonephritis.

117 Match the laboratory values with the appropriate disorder.
i. Na^+ 140 mmol/l, K^+ 2.5 mmol/l, $HCO3^-$ 18 mmol/l, urine pH 7.0, urine pCO_2 75 mmHg.
ii. Na^+ 140 mmol/l, K^+ 2.5 mmol/l, $HCO3^-$ 18 mmol/l, urine pH 7.0, urine pCO_2 50 mmHg.
iii. Na^+ 140 mmol/l, K^+ 2.5 mmol/l, $HCO3^-$ 15 mmol/l, urine pH 5.0, urine pCO_2 75 mmHg.
iv. Na^+ 140 mmol/l, K^+ 5.6 mmol/l, $HCO3^-$ 20 mmol/l, urine pH 5.0, urine pCO_2 75 mmHg.
(a) Type IV RTA.
(b) Type I (distal RTA).
(c) Type II (proximal RTA).
(d) Type I RTA (amphotericin-induced).

118 A 75-year-old man is admitted to the CCU with unstable angina. His regular medication includes warfarin. A coronary angiogram is performed the following day and the patient is discharged that evening. Three weeks later he returns to his physician complaining of nausea and cold painful feet (**118a**, courtesy of Drs Pai and Heywood, and *New England Journal of Medicine*). In contrast to his usual state he is confused and forgetful. Serum creatinine, which was previously normal, is now 5.9 mg/dl (520 µmol/l). A renal biopsy was undertaken (**118b**).

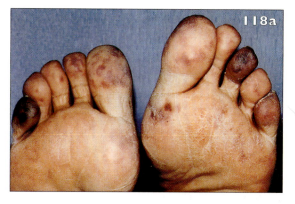

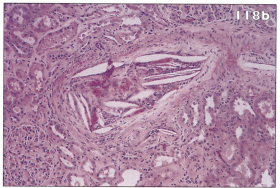

i. What has happened?
ii. What does the renal biopsy show?
iii. Could the diagnosis have been made in any other way?

Classification of Renal Tubule Acidification Defects

RTA	Urine pH	Plasma K$^+$	Urine pCO$_2$^{a}	Fanconi's	NH4$^+$
Type I	>5.5	Low	<70	No	Low
Type I (amphotericin-induced)	>5.5	Low	>70	No	Low
Type II	>variable^b	Low	>70	Frequent	Normal
Type IV	<5.5	High	>70	No	Low
Type I with distal hyperkalaemia	>5.5	High	>70	No	

^{a}With bicarbonate diuresis (mmHg) ^{b}Dependent upon serum [HCO$_3^-$]

117 i, (d); ii, (b); iii, (c); iv, (a) (see Table). Distal hypokalaemic RTA or Type I RTA is characterised by metabolic acidosis, an inability to maximally acidify the urine (urine pH >5.5), and hypokalaemia. The defect is thought to be secondary to H$^+$-ATP-ase dysfunction in the distal tubule. The cause of the hypokalaemia is not clear, but it may be secondary to acidosis-induced natriuresis, producing a hyperaldosterone state. If sufficient bicarbonate is delivered to the distal tubule, an intact proton pump should be able to raise the urinary pCO$_2$ to >70 mmHg by the reaction:

$$H^+ + HCO_3^- \Leftrightarrow H_2CO_3 \Leftrightarrow CO_2 + H_2O$$

If the H$^+$-ATP-ase does not function properly, urinary pCO$_2$ is <70 mmHg, a hallmark of Type I RTA, except in amphotericin-induced Type I RTA where the H$^+$-ATP-ase functions normally, but there is a 'back leak' of protons. This creates an inability to maximally acidify urine, but an ability to raise urine pCO$_2$ (i.e. >70 mmHg).

Type II RTA or proximal RTA is characterised by proximal bicarbonate wasting. Urinary pH is high as long as the serum bicarbonate is above the proximal tubule reabsorption threshold, whereas it is appropriately acidic (pH <5.5) when the serum bicarbonate is below this reabsorptive threshold. Hypokalaemia is common. Type II RTA is often accompanied by other features of Fanconi's syndrome.

Type IV RTA or hyporeninaemic hypoaldosteronism is characterised by hyperkalaemia and mild metabolic acidosis. Urinary pCO$_2$ is >70 mmHg and urine pH <5.5.

118 i. The patient has atheroembolic disease due to the angiogram catheter dislodging arteriosclerotic plaques showering atheroemboli downstream. Anticoagulation worsens the disease by preventing coverage of the damaged plaques with fibrin. As well as skin (118a) and mesenteric involvement, the kidneys are often affected.
ii. Cholesterol crystals are visible after tissue fixation as needle-shaped clear spaces (118b). Eosinophilia and decreased complement levels are common and, due to vascular occlusion, there is secondary glomerular sclerosis and progressive renal failure.
iii. The history and skin findings are so typical of atheroembolic disease that it is frequently possible to make the diagnosis without histological confirmation.

119 An elderly woman is admitted because of weakness, back pain and peripheral oedema. On admission, anaemia, thrombocytopenia, hypoalbuminaemia and renal insufficiency with nephrotic range proteinuria are present. Serum protein electrophoresis shows a monoclonal band with a concentration of 25 g/l. Her kidney biopsy is shown (**119**, courtesy of R. Hennigar, MD).

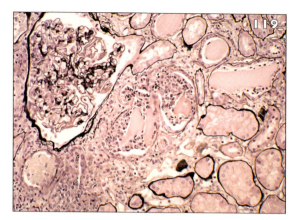

i. What is the most likely diagnosis?
ii. How would you confirm it?
iii. What is the treatment?

120 What is this (**120**) renal replacement therapy device, and what clinical advantages does it have?

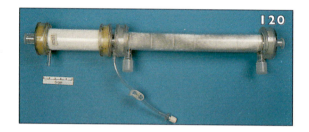

121 i. What abnormality is shown on this patient's back?
ii. What other skin lesions are frequently encountered in renal transplant recipients?
iii. What are some of the complications of CSA therapy?

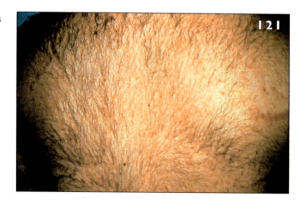

119 i. The tubules contain eosinophilic casts which are surrounded by a localised interstitial infiltrate. These features are suggestive of myeloma cast nephropathy.
ii. The diagnosis is confirmed by demonstrating the presence of >20% plasma cells or a monoclonal population of plasma cells in bone marrow biopsy. Tubular casts stain positively for the monoclonal protein. Under normal conditions, light chains are filtered, reabsorbed and metabolised by proximal tubular cells. When the proximal tubular capacity for reabsorption is exceeded, light chains coprecipitate with Tamm–Horsfall protein to form casts that obstruct the tubules. Disruption of the tubular basement membrane and localised interstitial inflammation ensues. Conditions that increase the concentration of light chains in the tubules, such as dehydration, diuretic use or proximal tubular injury, may potentiate cast formation. A pathogenetic role for light chains is suggested by the development of lesions in mice similar to cast nephropathy when light chains eluted from human myeloma kidneys are infused.
iii. Initial treatment should be directed at limiting further cast formation by avoiding dehydration or potentially nephrotoxic drugs and reversing hypercalcaemia. Chemotherapy is administered (e.g., melphalan plus prednisone) to reduce the paraprotein concentration, in the hope of preventing progression of renal failure. Plasmapheresis has been advocated to reduce the paraprotein concentration, but its benefit on renal recovery remains unproven. Despite treatment, the prognosis for patients with nephropathy is poor, with a median survival less than 2 years.

120 Shown is a combined haemodialyser and haemofilter unit. A hollow fibre cuprophane haemodialyser is combined with a high-flux haemofilter to provide increased solute removal by the combination of diffusive clearance (at the haemodialyser) and convective clearance (at the haemofilter). The technique, called paired filtration dialysis (PFD) achieves an increased total mass transfer in comparison with standard haemodialysis or haemodiafiltration (at comparable blood, dialysate and ultrafiltration rates), providing the opportunity to reduce treatment times. Additionally, better convective clearances improve middle molecule removal. Wide acceptance of the technique has been limited by the high cost of the combined device.

121 i. Hypertrichosis is shown, a complication of CSA. It is especially common in dark-skinned individuals, and typically produces thick pigmented hair on the trunk, back shoulders, arms, neck, forehead and cheeks.
ii. Other CSA complications include nephrotoxicity (acute and chronic), hyperkalaemia, hyperuricaemia, hypomagnesaemia, glucose intolerance, tremor, dysaesthesias, hypertension, hyperlipidaemia and gingival hypertrophy. More unusual complications of CSA include seizures, lymphomas, hepatotoxicity and haemolytic uraemic syndrome.

122 A 32-year-old man has a history of recurrent calcium oxalate nephrolithiasis. His first stone occurred at 25 years of age. There is no family history of nephrolithiasis. His examination is completely normal and an IVP shows linear striations in the papillae and occasional medullary cystic collections of contrast and calcium. A 24-hour urine collection while eating his usual diet is remarkable only for hypercalciuria [>400 mg/day (>10 mmol/day)]. His serum chemistries are given (Tables).

i. What type of kidney disease does this patient have and what is the acid–base abnormality?

ii. What therapy do you recommend?

Serum	Result
Sodium	139 mmol/l
Potassium	4.0 mmol/l
Chloride	109 mmol/l
Total CO_2	19 mmol/l
Creatinine	1.1 mmol/l (97 μmol/l)

Urine	Result
Urine pH	5.8

Arterial blood gas	Result
Arterial pH	7.37
Arterial pCO_2	34 mmHg

123 A 7-year-old boy had been seen in the emergency room on eight occasions during the previous year. He typically complains of the sudden onset of nausea, vomiting and abdominal pain. Within 2–3 hours the pain resolves spontaneously and urinalyses obtained during each evaluation have been normal. What does the IVP (**123**) show and how would you manage this patient?

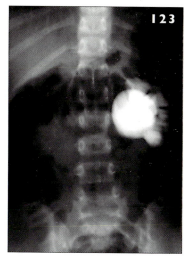

124 A 55-year-old man with ESRD secondary to hypertension on haemodialysis expresses concern to you about his risk of heart disease. He was a smoker until 2 years previously, has a strong family history for myocardial infarction and, on his recent monthly dialysis laboratories studies, had an elevated triglyceride level. His brother, who has no health problems other than isolated hypertriglyceridaemia, was recently started on clofibrate. The patient wonders if he should be taking this drug as well. What do you advise this patient?

122 i. He has medullary sponge kidney disease complicated by a normal anion-gap metabolic acidosis and hypercalciuria. Medullary sponge kidney disease is an autosomal recessive disease associated with dilated medullary collecting ducts. Nephrolithiasis occurs in up to 25% of patients with medullary sponge kidney disease and 50% have hypercalciuria. They often have haematuria and urinary tract infections, but renal failure is uncommon. Distal RTA (Type I) develops as a result of damage to the collecting ducts. Characteristic features include non-gap metabolic acidosis, inability to acidify the urine below pH 5.5, nephrolithiasis and a positive urinary anion gap.
ii. The metabolic acidosis is corrected with oral alkali therapy provided as bicarbonate or citrate salts. Sodium salts should be avoided because of the patient's history of hypercalciuria and nephrolithiasis. In addition, he should be encouraged to increase his fluid intake to achieve a urine output >2 l/day, to restrict dietary sodium (about 2 g/day) and protein (about 1 g protein/kg/day), and to start a thiazide diuretic. A urine collection should be repeated 4–8 weeks after starting therapy to confirm that the interventions had been successful in reducing hypercalciuria.

123 This is a common clinical presentation for a patient with a partial ureteropelvic junction obstruction, exacerbated by increased fluid intake. Since ultrasonography is non-invasive, it is usually performed initially to evaluate these patients. If hydronephrosis is confirmed, an IVP is then performed to delineate the site of obstruction. It is very important to evaluate these patients at the time of presentation, or after inducing diuresis with frusemide (furosemide), since hydronephrosis may resolve as the urine flow rate declines. A pyeloplasty is the procedure of choice for correcting ureteropelvic junction obstruction.

124 The patient should be advised that clofibrate is contraindicated in patients with renal insufficiency. Normally, the clofibrate metabolite, chlorophenoxyisobutyric acid, is conjugated with glucuronic acid and excreted by the kidney. When clofibrate is given in standard doses to patients with renal failure, chlorophenoxyisobutyric acid accumulates. In addition, uraemic patients deconjugate the glucuronide metabolite, resulting in even higher blood levels of chlorophenoxyisobutyric acid. High levels of chlorophenoxyisobutyric acid are associated with myopathy, rhabdomyolysis and hyperkalaemia.
The patient's concerns regarding his triglyceride levels should initially be addressed by recommencing weight reduction (if obese), a low-fat diet and exercise. If this fails to decrease lipid levels, small doses of lipid-lowering medications, such as gemfibrizol (for hypertriglyceridemia) or an HMG CoA-reductase inhibitor (for elevated LDL cholesterol) could be considered.

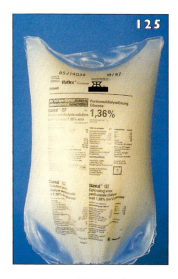

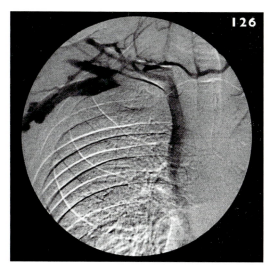

125 Shown (125) is the CAPD peritoneal effluent of a patient with suspected peritonitis.
i. How would you confirm the diagnosis?
ii. What is the most likely infecting organism?
iii. What treatment would you recommend?

126 This investigation (126) was undertaken in a haemodialysis patient who developed a swollen arm after construction of a brachial arteriovenous fistula.
i. What is the investigation and what does it show?
ii. How might this condition be treated?

127 The renal biopsy in 127 is from a patient with acute nephritic syndrome. What is the diagnosis?

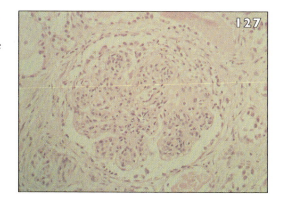

125 i. The diagnosis of peritonitis in a CAPD patient is made if two of the following are present: abdominal pain, a white cell count in dialysate >100/µl (>50% neutrophils), or the presence of micro-organisms in the effluent.

If infective peritonitis is suspected because of abdominal pain or cloudy dialysate, a Gram stain and cell count of the peritoneal fluid should be performed.

ii. At presentation the clinician should try to identify a reason for developing peritonitis, such as technique or equipment failure. Peritonitis usually occurs because of faulty technique or periluminar spread from an exit-site infection; thus *Staphylococci* (*albus* and *aureus*) are the most frequent infecting organisms. Culture-negative episodes usually reflect inadequacies in effluent collection and culture, but may point to an unusual infection, such as tuberculosis, where the effluent cell count may show a disproportionate number of monocytes. The clinician should also consider other surgical causes of abdominal pain, such as appendicitis, strangulated herniae or pancreatitis, before deciding that the patient has CAPD peritonitis.

iii. Most episodes of CAPD peritonitis will respond to antibiotic therapy. These may be administered intravenously; however, the intraperitoneal route is used most often. Mild cases may be treated by self administration of antibiotics as an out-patient. It is important to recognise the need for more intensive antibiotic therapy and early catheter removal in more severe cases. Prompt catheter removal will reduce morbidity and mortality following CAPD peritonitis and should be seriously considered for infections not resolving within 48 hours of treatment and for all cases of fungal peritonitis. Surgery may be required in selected cases where bowel perforation, abscess formation or other intra-abdominal pathology is suspected.

126 i. This is a venogram showing an occlusion of the subclavian vein at the mid-clavicular level, which has been caused by repeated cannulation of the subclavian vein for temporary vascular access. In some patients this does not present until the construction of an arteriovenous fistula increases the venous pressure, causing arm oedema.

ii. A stricture or partial occlusion can be treated by either stenting or balloon angioplasty. This not always successful and the stricture can recur.

127 This pattern is characteristic of post-infectious glomerulonephritis, which is most commonly post-streptococcal, but may be provoked by a wide range of infectious agents. Serum C3 is typically depressed and large deposits ('humps') of IgG and C3 are found along the glomerular capillary wall by immunofluorescence. Electron microscopy shows electron-dense deposits that correspond to the 'humps' on the subepithelial side of the glomerular basement membrane. The cells that fill the capillary loops are mostly neutrophils.

Despite the intense glomerular infiltration, rapid resolution is typical and usually leaves little or no residual glomerular scarring.

128 A 40-year-old woman presents with muscle twitching, cramps and paraesthesia. She has been receiving cisplatin and cyclophosphamide for ovarian cancer during the past several weeks. Despite receiving chemotherapy she has maintained a good oral intake and denies ethanol ingestion. Physical examination shows positive Chvostek and Trousseau signs. Muscle fasciculations are evident with percussion. Laboratory results show serum magnesium 1.2 mg/dl (0.5 mmol/l) and serum total calcium 6.0 mg/dl (1.5 mmol/l).
i. What is the cause of the patient's complaints?
ii. What is the aetiology of the changes in the magnesium and calcium concentrations?

129 An 18-year-old mentally retarded girl presented with a grand mal seizure. On examination a papular facial rash was noted (**129a**) and a blood pressure of 204/118 mmHg was recorded. Plasma creatinine was 150 μmol/l (1.7 mg/dl) and IVP was performed (**129b**).
i. Describe the skin changes seen in **129a**. What is the underlying condition and what are the other dermatological features?
ii. Describe the changes seen on the IVP. Would additional imaging provide further information?
iii. What other investigations would you perform?
iv. What is the inheritance of this condition?

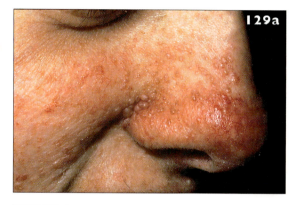

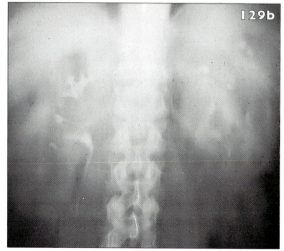

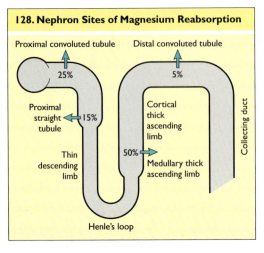

128. Nephron Sites of Magnesium Reabsorption

Proximal convoluted tubule — 25%

Distal convoluted tubule — 5%

Proximal straight tubule ← 15%

Thin descending limb

Cortical thick ascending limb

50% → Medullary thick ascending limb

Collecting duct

Henle's loop

128 i. The patient's symptoms and physical findings are a result of hypomagnesaemia and hypocalcaemia.

ii. Hypomagnesaemia is a frequent complication of cisplatin therapy occurring in approximately 50% of patients receiving this drug. Illustrated (**128**) are the sites of magnesium absorption in the nephron. Damage to these sites leads to renal magnesium wasting, possibly related to mitochondrial damage in these segments. The severity of cisplatin tubular damage is related to the dose and frequency of administration. The tubular defect usually resolves over several weeks if cisplatin therapy is withheld. However, in some instances renal magnesium wasting may persist for years. Other drugs which can induce renal magnesium wasting include aminoglycosides, diuretics and cyclosporin.

Hypocalcaemia can develop in severe cases of hypomagnesaemia because the low levels of magnesium lead to blunted release and decreased peripheral responsiveness to PTH. Correction of the magnesium deficit results in restoration of PTH to normal levels within several days.

Cisplatin nephrotoxicity can be minimised by vigorous hydration and diuresis during its administration and by avoiding cumulative doses over 120 mg/m^2 body surface area.

129 i. The skin changes are those of adenoma sebaceum, which is characteristic of tuberous sclerosis. The other dermatological features include hypomelanotic macules (shown with ultraviolet illumination) and a 'shagreen patch' over the back. Fibromas of the nail bed are also common.

ii. The IVP shows bilaterally enlarged kidneys with calyceal distortion due to multiple cysts. An ultrasound examination might show solid angiomyolipomas in addition to the cysts.

iii. A CT or MRI scan of the brain should be undertaken to identify tubers of the cerebral cortex. Retinal hamartomas (phakomas) may also be identified by funduscopy.

iv. Tuberous sclerosis is an autosomal dominant condition and loci have been identified on chromosomes 9 (TSC1) and 16 (TSC2). Approximately 80% of cases are sporadic. The gene product of TSC2, tuberin, has also been characterised.

130 A 65-year-old man, on peritoneal dialysis for 8 years, presents with acute peritonitis. After 48 hours of antibiotic therapy, the patient is asymptomatic. An ultrasound was ordered to exclude an intra-abdominal abscess, but it reveals small atrophic kidneys with multiple bilateral small simple cysts, and one 3 cm right renal cyst with internal echos. A CT scan confirms that the latter cyst is complex with an irregular border, internal debris and haemorrhage. At surgery a renal cell carcinoma was found in this complex cyst and a nephrectomy was performed. Which of the following is the patient most likely to have?

i. Medullary cystic disease with malignant transformation.
ii. ARPKD with malignant transformation.
iii. Acquired renal cystic disease with malignant transformation.
iv. ADPKD with malignant transformation.

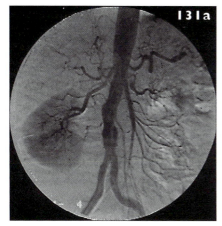

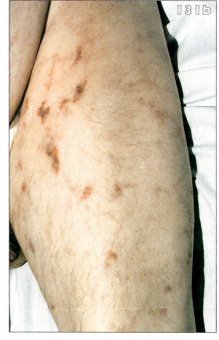

131 A 63-year-old man with peripheral vascular disease, ischaemic heart disease and long-standing hypertension developed deteriorating blood pressure control and plasma creatinine increased from 1.1 mg/dl (96 μmol/l) to 2.6 mg/dl (230 μmol/l) over 6 months. An angiogram was performed (131a), and 2 weeks later he developed a lower extremity rash (131b).

i. Why was the angiogram performed and what does it show?
ii. What is the skin rash most likely due to?

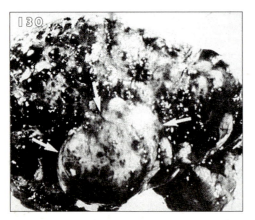

130 iii. The diagnosis is established in the proper setting (i.e., chronic renal failure with no family history of polycystic kidney disease) by documenting four or more bilateral cysts (usually <0.5 cm in diameter) in small- to normal-sized, smoothly surfaced kidneys. Unlike polycystic kidney disease, extrarenal cysts are not observed in acquired renal cystic disease. Multiple simple renal cysts are observed in 7% of predialysis chronic renal failure patients, with the incidence increasing to 22% of dialysis patients. Of patients on dialysis for more than 10 years, 50–80% will develop acquired renal cystic disease. White women have the lowest risk while black men are at the highest risk for developing acquired renal cystic disease.

While cyst haemorrhage may occur in up to 50% of cases, pain and haematuria are uncommon. The incidence of malignant transformation of acquired cysts is 4–7%. However, the incidence of renal cell carcinoma in the ESRD population (1–3%) is only slightly higher than in the general population. Recommendations for screening the ESRD population for acquired cystic disease vary. Some experts recommend that after 3–5 years of dialysis, renal ultrasounds be performed annually. Others suggest routine screening be withheld until haematuria, flank pain or long dialysis durations (>5–10 years) occur. Suspicious cysts greater than 2–3 cm in diameter, or increasing in size on serial imaging, should be surgically removed. Bilateral nephrectomy is preferred since the carcinomas may be multiple and bilateral. A gross specimen of a renal cell carcinoma in a patient with acquired renal cystic disease is shown (130).

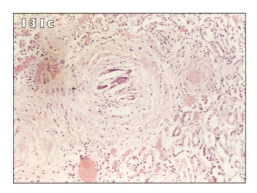

131 i. The angiogram was performed because deteriorating renal function and blood pressure control in a patient with peripheral vascular disease suggests the possibility of atherosclerotic renovascular disease. 131a shows irregularity of the lower aorta and common iliac vessels due to atheroma. There is a stenosis at the origin of both renal arteries.
ii. The skin rash is probably due to atheroemboli (131c).

132 A 33-year-old woman with a history of ulcerative colitis is admitted to the hospital for an exacerbation of her inflammatory bowel disease. Laboratory data are Na^+ 135 mmol/l, K^+ 3.8 mmol/l, Cl^- 110 mmol/l, HCO_3^- 14 mmol/l, BUN 19 mg/dl (6.8 mmol/l), creatinine 1.5 mg/dl (133 µmol/l); ABG, pH 7.21, pCO_2 22 mmHg, pO_2 95 mmHg; and urine Na^+ 38 mmol/l, K^+ 42 mmol/l, Cl^- 65 mmol/l and pH 5.0.
i. What is this patient's urinary anion gap?
ii. Is this patient's metabolic acidosis solely from diarrhoea or is there also a renal acidification defect?

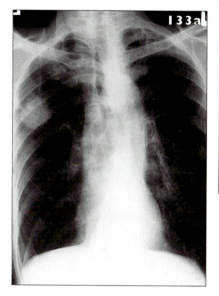

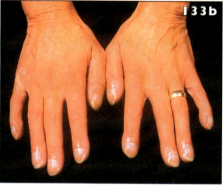

133 This 72-year-old man has nephrotic syndrome.
i. What is the likely explanation for the chest radiograph (**133a**) appearance?
ii. What is the most likely finding on renal biopsy?

134 A 26-year-old woman was found to have a blood pressure of 204/118 mmHg at a routine medical examination. She was referred for investigation and a renal angiogram was performed (**134**).
i. What does the angiogram show?
ii. What is the likely aetiology of this?
iii. What is the natural history of this condition?
iv. What is the relationship between this condition and the hypertension?

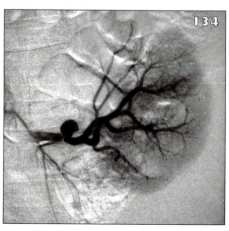

132 i. Net acid excretion by the kidney is equal to NH_4^+ plus titratable acids minus HCO_3^-. In the face of an increased acid load or bicarbonate loss, the kidney will excrete a larger amount of NH_4^+ (ammonium). Thus, the urinary anion gap, i.e., $Na^+ + K^+ - Cl^-$, will be negative if the kidney is appropriately generating NH_4^+ in response to the metabolic acidosis induced by gastrointestinal bicarbonate losses. In this patient, the urinary anion gap is $38 + 42 - 65 = +15$.
ii. As the urinary anion gap is positive, this indicates that renal ammonium excretion is impaired and that a renal acidification defect is present. Note the urinary anion gap gives no clue as to the nature of the defect.

133 i. Carcinoma of the bronchus.
ii. Membranous nephropathy, which is associated with malignancy, most typically carcinoma. It is an unusual association – only about 2% of patients with membranous nephropathy are found to have malignancy either before or after the renal disease presents. This may be an underestimate as patients with oedema may not be assessed in detail in the context of advanced malignancy. However, 'blind' investigation for malignancy in patients with membranous nephropathy is not recommended, although suspicious clinical symptoms and signs should be fully assessed.

134 i. The angiogram shows a saccular aneurysm of the renal artery with a proximal stenosis. The upper pole of the kidney appears to be poorly perfused.
ii. Both of these abnormalities are common features of fibromuscular dysplasia.
iii. In fibromuscular dysplasia renal artery stenosis is less likely to proceed to complete occlusion of the artery than in the atheromatous form. The aneurysm is unlikely to rupture unless it exceeds 2 cm. However, in pregnancy there is an increased risk of rupture and if the patient was planning a pregnancy then occlusion of the aneurysm could be attempted by inserting a spring coil into the lumen.
iv. In renal artery stenosis hypertension develops because of increased renin release in response to decreased perfusion. A renal artery aneurysm in the absence of a stenosis can by itself be associated with hypertension, because of either a decrease in distal flow or through thrombotic emboli.

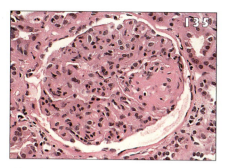

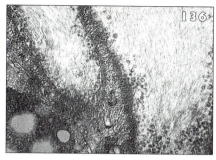

135 A 34-year-old black man developed ESRD secondary to focal segmental glomerulosclerosis (FSGS). The time from detection of nephrotic range proteinuria to ESRD was 12 months. After 2 years on chronic haemodialysis, he underwent cadaveric renal transplantation. Nephrotic range proteinuria recurred 6 months later, and a renal biopsy was obtained (**135**, courtesy of R. Hennigar, MD).
i. What does the biopsy demonstrate?
ii. What therapy is appropriate?

136 An elderly man with congestive heart failure and peripheral neuropathy is referred because of progressive renal insufficiency and nephrotic syndrome. A kidney biopsy shows acellular material filling the mesangium, which was Congo red positive. An EM image of a deposit is shown (**136**). What is the diagnosis?

137 Shown (**137**) is the growth chart of a 10-year-old boy treated with CAPD for 3 years.
i. Which form of renal replacement therapy optimises growth in children with renal failure?
ii. What other factors influence growth in children with end-stage renal failure?

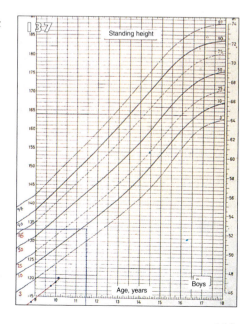

113

135 i. The renal biopsy demonstrates recurrent FSGS. This entity recurs in approximately one-third of patients and leads to graft failure in 50%. The recurrence rate is highest in patients for whom the original disease was very aggressive, such as the case presented here.

ii. Therapy for recurrent FSGS has been as disappointing, as that seen with primary FSGS. Neither CSA nor FK506 have appreciably attenuated the course of recurrent FSGS compared with previous experience using azathioprine. There are a few reports of short-term success with multiple courses of plasma exchange. Such therapies are directed towards reducing the putative humoral factor(s) at play in this disease. Repeat renal transplantation should be considered cautiously since the recurrence rate in such patients is greater than 80%.

136 EM demonstrates non-branching fibrils of variable length, measuring less than 10 nm in diameter. The combination of Congo red positivity and narrow non-branching fibrils is diagnostic of amyloidosis.

The *fibrillary glomerulopathies* are characterised by extracellular deposition of microfibrils. Congo red birefringence differentiates *amyloid* (positive Congo red birefringence) from *non-amyloid* filbrillary glomerulopathies.

In amyloidosis a variety of proteins (AL, SAA,) are able to polymerise in a beta-pleated sheet pattern, with apple-green birefringence under polarising light using the Congo red stain. In non-amyloid glomerulopathies, a deposited immunoglobulin (or immunoglobulin fragment) can be detected by immunofluorescence using specific antibodies. Conditions associated with non-amyloid glomerulopathies include *cryoglobulinaemia* and *monoclonal gammopathies* (either benign monoclonal gammopathies or associated with multiple myeloma). *Immunotactoid glomerulopathy* is a recently described entity. The precise composition of the fibrils is not known, although both heavy and light chains and amyloid P component are present. Involvement is restricted to the glomerulus, and it does not result in a multisystem disease. Response to therapy is poor, with 50% progressing to end-stage renal failure in 2–4 years.

137 i. This patient's height is below the 3rd centile at the start of CAPD and on dialysis his growth remains parallel to, but below, the 3rd centile. It is usually accepted that growth potential is best achieved by early successful transplantation using corticosteroid-sparing immunosuppression regimes. Growth may be better on CAPD than haemodialysis but, as in this case, catch-up growth is usually not seen.

ii. Growth may be maximised in children undergoing dialysis by optimising nutrition and dialysis adequacy, and by correcting acid–base disturbance and renal osteodystrophy. The use of exogenous growth hormone therapy can overcome growth retardation, especially in the first 2 years of treatment. However, its value in the longer term is yet to be established.

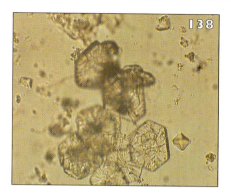

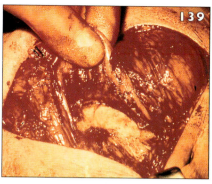

138 A 26-year-old woman complains of nausea, vomiting, severe right flank pain radiating to her groin and dark urine. She has no personal or family history of kidney disease, takes no medications and follows no specific dietary restrictions. Her blood pressure is 140/90 mmHg, heart rate 100 b.p.m., temperature 37.2°C and weight 60 kg. She had right loin tenderness, but her physical examination was otherwise normal. Her serum electrolytes, urea nitrogen, creatinine, calcium and uric acid were normal. An IVP showed a radiopaque filling defect in the right ureter with partial obstruction. Urine microscopy was undertaken and the results shown in 138.
i. What is the cause of her pain?
ii. What studies would you recommend to evaluate her problem?
iii. What therapy would you prescribe?

139 i. This CAPD patient is undergoing a laparotomy. What is shown in 139?
ii. What is the treatment?

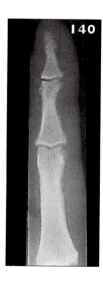

140 Shown (140) is a radiograph of the first finger of a haemodialysis patient who has been complaining of increasing musculoskeletal pain.
i. What does the radiograph show?
ii. What is the abnormality and pathogenesis of this condition?

138 i. The hexagonal crystals shown (**138**) are characteristic of cystine. Cystinuria is a rare cause of nephrolithiasis resulting from a defect in proximal tubule cystine transport. It is an autosomal recessive disorder and patients typically begin forming stones between the first and fourth decades. Cystine stones are radiopaque and can form staghorn calculi.

ii. Cystinuria is confirmed by documenting an increase in 24-hour urinary cystine excretion. Normal excretion is about 10–100 mg/day (40–420 μmol/day) whereas patients with cystinuria excrete more than 400 mg/day (1.6 mmol/day). Stones form because cystine has limited solubility [300 mg/l (1.2 mmol/l)].

iii. Therapy is directed at maintaining cystine in solution. This can be achieved by increasing urine volume (i.e., >3 l/day) and alkalinising the urine which increases cystine solubility. In severe cases, penicillamine and captopril have been used as adjuvant therapy. Penicillamine complexes with cysteine, thereby preventing crystallisation. Unfortunately, the adverse side-effects of penicillamine limit its use. Captopril appears to be a promising therapy; its sulphhydryl groups complex with cysteine, thus decreasing cystinuria. Cystine stones are resistant to extracorporeal shock-wave lithotripsy.

139 i. The patient has sclerosing peritonitis, a rare condition the incidence of which has decreased in recent years. The surgeon's fingers (**139**) are holding a sheath of new fibrous tissue which is encapsulating the contents of the peritoneal cavity, causing small bowel obstruction. The condition often presents with weight loss, anorexia, vomiting and bowel obstruction. The diagnosis is usually made, as in this case, at laparotomy, but may be suspected by barium follow through and abdominal ultrasound examinations.

ii. Sclerosing peritonitis results from excessive fibrosis, which is thought to be an idiosyncratic reaction of the peritoneum to a variety of irritant factors. Acetate dialysate and chlorhexidine antiseptic have been abandoned because of their association with sclerosing peritonitis. There is no known effective treatment for the condition. Surgery should be reserved for selected cases with bowel obstruction; the role of immunosuppressive therapy, which has been reported to be beneficial in some patients, remains to be clarified.

140 i. The radiograph (**140**) shows subperiosteal erosions and loss of the tuft of the terminal phalanx.

ii. These changes are characteristic of hyperparathyroidism, but they are often a late feature of this complication of chronic renal failure (CRF) and their absence does not rule out hyperparathyroidism. Measurement of iPTH is a sensitive method of diagnosing hyperparathyroidism. The increased synthesis and release of PTH in CRF results from several factors, including low levels of 1,25-dihydroxyvitamin D_3, low concentrations of ionised calcium and increased serum phosphate levels. Normally 1,25-dihydroxyvitamin D_3 directly suppresses the synthesis of PTH.

141 This urine sample (**141**) was taken from a 23-year-old woman who presented with a febrile illness, vomiting and left loin pain.
i. What is this abnormality?
ii. What is the explanation for the patient's illness?
iii. What other conditions can cause this urinary appearance?

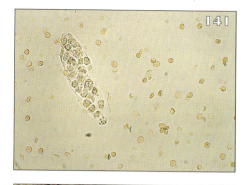

142 A 37-year-old man with ESRD secondary to hypertension received a mismatched cadaveric renal transplant 5 years ago. His post-operative course was complicated by one episode of acute rejection and he has been maintained on a regimen of prednisone 10 mg/day, azathioprine 100 mg/day and CSA 2 mg/kg/day. For the past year his serum creatinine has gradually increased from 1.8 mg/dl (160 μmol/l) to 2.4 mg/dl

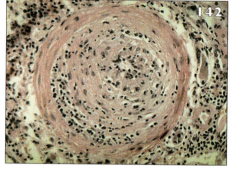

(212 μmol/l) and a 24-hour urine collection reveals 1.7 g/day of protein. A renal biopsy was performed (**142**).
i. What does the biopsy show?
ii. How should this patient be treated?

143 A 79-year-old woman developed massive bruising of the left groin following an unsuccessful attempt to position a left femoral vein haemodialysis catheter. The results of an investigative procedure are shown in **143**.
i. What is this investigation?
ii. What abnormality of the left femoral artery does it demonstrate?

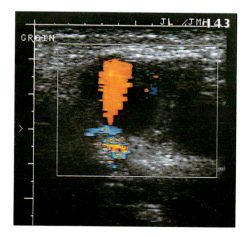

141 i. This is a white cell cast.
ii. This patient was suffering from acute pyelonephritis. The presence of very occasional leucocytes in the urine may occur in healthy individuals, but high numbers most commonly reflect urinary infection. The presence of white cell casts in the urine indicates renal parenchymal involvement. A mid-stream specimen should be sent for Gram's stain and bacteriological culture to assist in antibiotic selection.
iii. White cell casts should be expected in any condition characterised by a leucocyte infiltration of the renal interstitium. Whereas polymorph-containing white cell casts suggest acute pyelonephritis, lymphocyte casts are seen in allergic (drug-induced) interstitial nephritis (AIN), acute renal transplant rejection and lymphomatous infiltration of the kidneys. The presence of eosinophils in the urine and within white cell casts supports a diagnosis of AIN, but also occurs in cholesterol embolisation to the kidneys, and Churg–Strauss vasculitis. Identification of different leucocytes and, indeed, distinguishing leucocytes from tubular cells may be difficult with light microscopy. Laboratory staining techniques and phase-contrast microscopy may be of assistance in this situation.

Although the finding of white cell casts in urine strongly suggests renal interstitial disease, they may also occur in glomerulonephritis. Other urinary abnormalities, such as erythrocytes, red cell casts and granular casts would, however, be expected with this diagnosis.

142 i. The biopsy demonstrates proliferative vasculopathy, one of the hallmarks of chronic allograft rejection. Other features include tubulointerstitial fibrosis and glomerular sclerosis. The mechanisms responsible for this chronic, progressive nephropathy are unknown and an area of intense research. An immunological component is likely, given the association with HLA mismatching, prior episodes of acute rejection and insufficient doses of CSA. Non-immunological factors and non-specific inflammatory mediators postulated in other forms of progressive renal injury are also likely to contribute.
ii. To date, no therapy has proved beneficial. The best treatment is prevention by close follow-up and maintenance of adequate immunosuppression. Efforts to address non-immunological factors which may contribute to progressive injury are also appropriate. For example, hypertension is commonly present and inadequate control is associated with accelerated deterioration in graft function, so careful attention to blood pressure control is important. Similarly, hyperlipidaemia is commonly present, so lipid-lowering agents may be beneficial. Short-term studies of low-protein diets also suggest limited efficacy in slowing the rate of decline in renal function.

143 i. This is a colour Doppler ultrasound of the patient's left femoral artery.
ii. The study demonstrates a false aneurysm of the femoral artery. The jet of arterial blood (orange) is clearly seen entering the lumen of the false aneurysm. This unusual traumatic complication of femoral cannulation can normally be treated by prolonged manual pressure over the site of abnormality.

144 A 24-year-old student presented with a 7-day history of headache and vomiting. His blood pressure was found to vary between 150/90 and 210/130 mmHg. A 24-hour urine collection for catecholamines gave adrenaline (epinephrine) 1169 ng/24h (normal 20–190 ng/24h), noradrenaline (norepinephrine) 4396 ng/24h (normal 90–600 ng/24h). An abdominal CT scan was undertaken (144).

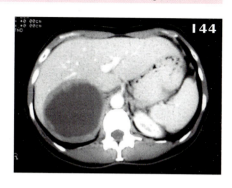

i. What is the significance of the urinary catecholamine results?
ii. Are additional biochemical investigations necessary and if so which ones?
iii. What abnormalities are seen on the CT scan?
iv. How should the patient be treated?

145 A 24-year-old diabetic received a one-haplotype matched renal transplant from her sibling 3 months previously. One month ago, she underwent a 14-day course of OKT3 for biopsy-proven severe rejection. Two days ago she reported the onset of fevers and allograft tenderness. Her serum creatinine was unchanged at 1.3 mg/dl (115 μmol/l), and her urinalysis demonstrated trace proteinuria and no pyuria. A renal biopsy was obtained (145). What is the best course of therapy?

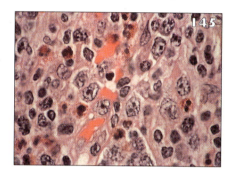

146 A 45-year-old hypertensive woman treated with thiazide diuretics complains of a 3-day history of anorexia and diarrhoea. She denied fever, abdominal pain, haematochezia or melena. On physical examination there was a 30 mmHg orthostatic change in blood pressure, hyperactive bowel sounds, watery haemoccult-negative stool and a soft abdomen. Her laboratory studies are given (Table).

Serum	Value
Sodium	140 mmol/l
Potassium	3.5 mmol/l
Chloride	96 mmol/l
Total CO_2	32 mmol/l
Creatinine	1.4 mg/dl (124 μmol/l)
Urea nitrogen	40 mg/dl (14 mmol/l)
Uric acid	10.5 mg/dl (624 μmol/l)

i. What are the possible causes of her hyperuricaemia?
ii. What therapy should be instituted?

144 i. The urinary catecholamine results are suggestive of a phaeochromocytoma.
ii. Twofold elevation above the normal range is considered diagnostic and in this case one 24-hour urine collection is sufficient. However, adrenaline (epinephrine) and noradrenaline (norepinephrine) secretion is episodic and at least two 24-hour collections should be undertaken. That adrenaline is increased as well as noradrenaline suggests that the tumour is in the adrenal gland. This is because the enzyme responsible for the conversion of noradrenaline into adrenaline, noradrenaline N-methyltransferase, is present only in the adrenal gland. Additional biochemical investigations are not necessary in the presence of such unequivocal changes.
iii. The CT scan shows a right adrenal mass.
iv. Treatment should be instituted initially with the non-selective alpha-blocker phenoxybenzamine followed by a beta-blocker. After adequate medical blockade the phaeochromocytoma should be removed surgically.

145 The biopsy reveals lymphocytes infiltrating the interstitium. This lesion should not be mistaken for acute rejection as it is, in fact, a lymphoproliferative process secondary to infection with Ebstein–Barr virus (EBV). EBV infection has often been implicated (although not exclusively) in the pathogenesis of a spectrum of diseases classified as post-transplant lymphoproliferative disease. The severity of illness ranges from a self-limited mononucleosis-like syndrome to malignant lymphoma. Primary EBV infection and one or more intensive courses of immunosuppression, such as the OKT3 given to this patient, have been implicated as factors that contribute to the expression of this potentially fatal disease. Appropriate therapy may include reduction and/or cessation of immunosuppression, surgical debulking or chemotherapy. The latter approach is reserved for advanced malignancies, although the response rate is poor, with up to 80% mortality.

146 i. The patient most likely has hyperuricaemia due to decreased excretion secondary to volume depletion from diarrhoea and thiazide diuretics. Hyperuricaemia occurs either because there is increased production or decreased renal excretion. Increased production occurs following cellular destruction (e.g., tumour lysis following chemotherapy) or high metabolic turnover (e.g., polycythaemia vera). Normally, urate is filtered, reabsorbed, secreted and then re-reabsorbed by the proximal tubule. Only 6–12% of the filtered urate is excreted. In volume-depleted states, there is increased proximal tubular urate reabsorption.
ii. Initially, the diuretic should be discontinued and her volume depletion corrected. Asymptomatic hyperuricaemia usually requires no pharmacological therapy.

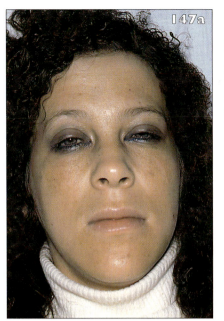 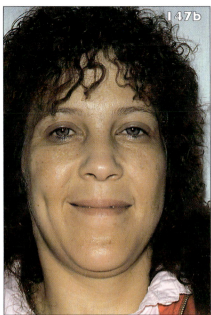

147 This 29-year-old patient felt ill within 5 minutes of commencing a haemodialysis session using a cuprophane dialysis membrane. She complained of chest tightness and dyspnoea and, on examination, was noted to have marked facial oedema (**147a**), bronchospasm and mild hypotension. Haemodialysis was discontinued, and she recovered with supportive therapy. **147b** shows her facial appearance the following day, having made a full recovery.
i. Explain this well-recognised complication of haemodialysis treatment.
ii. What treatment options are available?

148 A young woman is seen in the emergency department complaining of generalised weakness; she denies taking any medications. Her laboratory values show sodium 140 mmol/l, potassium 2.2 mmol/l, chloride 110 mmol/l, bicarbonate 27 mmo/l, BUN 16 mg/dl (5.7 mmol/l) and creatinine 1.0 mg/dl (88 μmol/l). Urine electrolytes are sodium 26 mmo/l, chloride 82 mmo/l and potassium 40 mmol/l. Her blood pressure is 120/70 mmHg. Which of the following are possible aetiologies of her hypokalaemia?
i. Surreptitious vomiting.
ii. Diuretic abuse.
iii. Bartter's syndrome.
iv. Primary hyperaldosteronism.

147 i. This patient experienced a dialyser reaction. Dialyser reactions can be divided into two types. This patient experienced a Type A (anaphylactic) reaction. Patients typically experience a burning heat sensation, angio-oedema, dyspnoea, urticaria, pruritus, rhinorrhoea, lacrimation and abdominal cramps within minutes of commencing haemodialysis treatment. Patients with a history of atopy are particularly prone to this complication.

Type A dialyser reactions are usually caused by hypersensitivity to ethylene oxide (ETO), which is used to sterilise hollow fibre dialysers. Elevated IgE antibody titres to ETO may be detected in the serum of such patients. The risk of ETO reaction is significantly reduced by carefully rinsing the dialyser before treatment is started. Similar anaphylactic reactions have been reported in patients dialysed with AN69 membrane while taking ACEI therapy. The reactions are thought to be mediated by the bradykinin system. Clinically indistinguishable reactions have also been attributed to heparin allergy. Re-used dialysers can be associated with Type A reactions because of endotoxin contamination of water used in the re-use process or failure to remove sterilant (formaldehyde, glutaraldehyde) from the dialysers before commencement of dialysis.

Type B dialyser reactions are more common and less severe. Typical symptoms are back and chest pain developing during the first hour of haemodialysis. The aetiology is uncertain, but may be related to complement activation resulting from the blood–membrane interaction.

ii. Patients with a history of a Type A reaction should avoid ETO-sterilised dialysers, and instead be treated with either steam-sterilised or gamma-irradiated dialysers. Treatment of an established reaction involves immediate termination of haemodialysis, without return of blood to the patient, and the administration of antihistamines, adrenaline (epinephrine) and/or corticosteroid therapy.

Patients with Type B reactions should use a dialysis membrane with less potential for complement activation, such as polysulphone.

148 ii, iii. It is very difficult clinically to distinguish surreptitious diuretic abuse and Bartter's syndrome. Both are manifested by a hypochloraemic, hypokalaemic metabolic alkalosis with a high urinary chloride (see table). In addition, both can be accompanied by hypomagnesaemia. A urine drug screen for diuretics is useful to confirm surreptitious diuretic abuse, which is much more common than Bartter's syndrome. Primary hyperaldosteronism is almost always accompanied by hypertension. Vomiting should produce a low urinary chloride.

Algorithm for Hypokalaemic Metabolic Alkalosis

Condition	Hypertension	Urinary Cl⁻	Urinary Na⁺
Primary aldosteronism	Yes	High	Variable
Vomiting	No	Low	Low
Bartter's syndrome	No	High	High/Variable
Diuretics	No	High	High
Secondary hyperaldosteronism	No	High	Low

149 A 28-year-old woman with hypertension is known to have cerebellar and retinal haemangioblastomas. For which of these secondary causes of hypertension should she be evaluated?
i. Primary aldosteronism.
ii. Coarctation of the aorta.
iii. Phaeochromocytoma.
iv. Renovascular stenosis.
v. Cushing's syndrome.

150 A 14-year-old girl is seen at a school medical examination. Her blood pressure is found to be 160/100 mmHg, weight 70 kg and height 1.47 m (4ft 10in). She is referred for further investigation. A chest radiograph (**150a**) and IVP (**150b**) are undertaken.
i. What abnormalities are seen on the chest radiograph?
ii. What are they due to?
iii. What abnormalities are seen on the IVP (**150b**)?
iv. What other clinical features would suggest a unifying diagnosis?
v. How should the hypertension be managed?

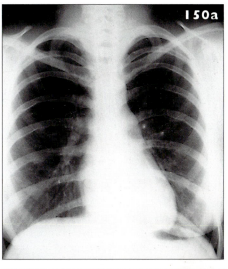

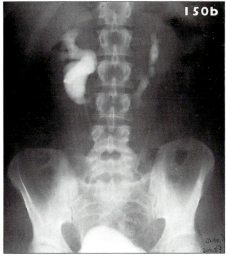

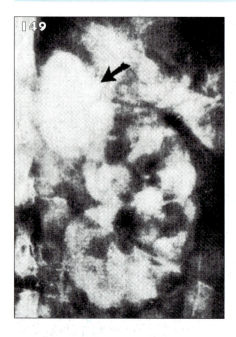

149 iii. Phaeochromocytoma. Von Hippel–Lindau syndrome is an autosomal dominant disease characterised by cerebellar and retinal haemangioblastomas, phaeochromocytomas and pancreatic and renal masses. The von Hippel–Lindau gene is located on chromosome 3, in a region which is frequently deleted in sporadic cases of renal cell carcinoma.

Phaeochromocytoma develops in 10–19% of patients with von Hippel–Lindau syndrome. Conversely, 20% of phaeochromocytoma patients are carriers for the von Hippel–Lindau gene. Renal cysts (**149**) and angiomas develop in 40–65% of von Hippel–Lindau patients. Mutations of the von Hippel–Lindau gene predispose to malignant degeneration. Although renal cell carcinoma is uncommon in patients <20 years old, about 70% of patients who survive to 60 years of age develop renal malignancy. Annual renal ultrasound screening is recommended for patients over the age of 20 years. CT is a more sensitive screening modality than renal ultrasound and has the advantage of also detecting adrenal adenomas.

150 i. The chest radiograph (**150a**) shows the heart size to be at the upper limit of normal and the mediastinum is slightly widened due to enlargement of the left subclavian artery. There is notching of the lower edge of the ribs.
ii. These features suggest a diagnosis of coarctation of the aorta.
iii. The IVU (IVP) (**150b**) shows that the lower poles of both kidneys are medial to the ureters. The right kidney is malrotated, characteristic of a horseshoe kidney. Horseshoe kidney by itself does not cause hypertension, but there are sometimes associated abnormalities of the renal artery.
iv. The combination of coarctation of the aorta and horseshoe kidney suggests an underlying diagnosis of Turner's syndrome – the girl's short stature is in keeping with this. Other features include a webbed neck, short fourth metacarpals, increased carrying angle of the arm, low-set ears, pigmented naevi, micronychia and epicanthic folds.
v. Coarctation should be treated in childhood because delayed correction does not cure hypertension. Surgical resection is safe with a low operative mortality. Angioplasty is a more recent approach and is sometimes reserved for recoarctation following surgical repair.

151 An elderly woman with long-standing rheumatoid arthritis (RA) treated with an oral gold preparation is referred because of progressive oedema. Physical examination is notable for hypertension, peripheral oedema and articular changes compatible with RA. Abnormal laboratory values include serum creatinine 1.8 mg/dl (160 μmol/l), serum albumin 22 g/l, total protein 76 g/l; urinalysis, 4+ protein, 1+ blood, negative glucose, 5–10 RBCs (HPF), occasional WBC and 2+ granular casts. A kidney biopsy is shown [**151a**, PAS stain and **151b**, Congo red stain (courtesy of R. Hennigar, MD)]. What is the diagnosis?

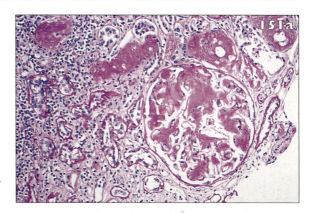

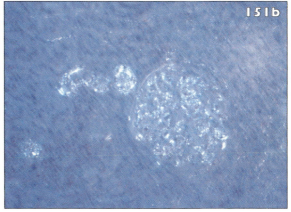

152 A 78-year-old black man complains of urinary frequency. His past medical history is significant for benign prostatic hypertrophy for 10 years. He has had two TURP procedures. A Foley catheter is placed after the patient attempted to urinate and the post-void residual is 300 ml. The patient appears well, blood pressure is 140/90 mmHg. Laboratory data are Na^+ 140 mmol/l, K^+ 6.1 mmol/l, Cl^- 112 mmol/l, HCO_3^- 20 mmol/l, BUN 31 mg/dl (11 mmol/l), creatinine 1.8 mg/dl (160 μmol/l), glucose 77 mg/dl (4.2 mmol/l) and urine pH 7.0. He has no history of diabetes and takes no medications. Which of the following is the most likely reason for his hyperkalaemia?

i. Type IV RTA.
ii. High potassium intake with renal insufficiency.
iii. Obstruction uropathy with distal (Type I) RTA.
iv. Adrenal insufficiency.

151 151a shows a large deposit of amorphous, acellular material filling the mesangium and extending into glomerular capillary loops. Nearby blood vessels are also involved. The apple-green birefringence under polarised light demonstrated by Congo red stain (**151b**) is diagnostic of amyloid. Based on the type of amyloid protein deposited, amyloidosis is classified as primary or secondary.

In *primary amyloidosis*, a variable region of immunoglobulin light chains (AL) is deposited, which is associated with a monoclonal proliferation of plasma cells. Multiple organ involvement is common and diagnosis is made by biopsy of the kidney or other affected organ. Approximately 20% of patients respond to prednisone and melphalan, but the long-term prognosis is poor with a 5-year survival of only 20%. In *secondary amyloidosis*, the breakdown products of an acute phase protein, serum amyloid A (SSA), are deposited in tissues. A variety of chronic inflammatory processes are associated with this form. RA, inflammatory bowel disease and chronic infections are the most common predisposing conditions. Familial Mediterranean fever (FMF) is a form of secondary amyloidosis which is inherited in an autosomal recessive pattern and occurs primarily in Sephardic Jews and people of Middle Eastern and Mediterranean origin. The treatment of secondary amyloidosis is directed at the underlying disease. In FMF, colchicine prevents recurrence of attacks and may slow the deposition of amyloid. A unique type of amyloidosis has been described in patients who receive long-term haemodialysis (>10 years); it is associated with the deposition of beta$_2$-microglobulin (B2M). Dialysis-associated amyloidosis most commonly involves the skeleton and results in a destructive arthropathy and carpal tunnel syndrome. Visceral involvement is rare. Following renal transplantation, serum B2M levels decrease, radiological improvement is observed and symptoms decline, presumably related to enhanced renal clearance of B2M.

152 iii. Chronic obstruction can cause a distal hyperkalaemic RTA. The hallmark of this condition is a distal potassium secretory defect along with an inability to maximally acidify the urine. Type IV RTA or 'hyporeninemic hypoaldosteronism' is most commonly seen in diabetics and usually does not impair maximal acidification of the urine. Adrenal insufficiency is usually accompanied by hypotension and should not interfere with maximal acidification. With this level of renal function, the kidney should be able to excrete potassium as long as no other tubular or hormonal defects are present.

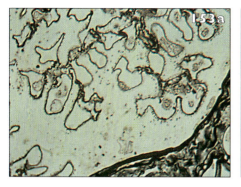 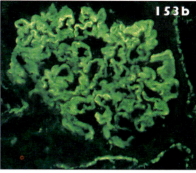

153 **153a** and **153b** are from the renal biopsy of a 60-year-old man who presented with nephrotic syndrome. What is the diagnosis?

154 Two years following cadaveric renal transplant a patient develops nephrotic-range proteinuria (3.6 g/24 h) and a gradually increasing serum creatinine. The patient states that he had a native kidney biopsy many years ago and was told he had 'glomerulonephritis'.
i. Would recurrent renal disease be possible in this patient?
ii. What does the biopsy (**154**) indicate?

155 A patient with a 2-week history of diarrhoea is admitted to the hospital. Laboratory tests show Na^+ 135 mmol/l, K^+ 2.5 mmol/l, HCO_3^- 19 mmol/l, BUN 25 mg/dl (8.9 mmol/l) and creatinine 1.6 mg/dl (142 μmol/l). Urinary electrolytes show sodium 15 mmol/l and potassium 20 mmol/l. Serum and urine osmolarity are 300 and 600 mOsm/l, respectively.
i. What is this patient's transtubular potassium gradient (TTKG)?
ii. Is this patient wasting or appropriately conserving potassium?

153 The diagnosis is membranous nephropathy. Methenamine silver stain (**153a**) shows 'spikes' on the outer surface of the glomerular capillary wall. These 'spikes' are new glomerular basement membrane developing between the granular deposits of IgG and C3, seen with immunofluorescence (**153b**). The immune deposits also appear as subepithelial electron dense deposits on EM. The majority of patients have *idiopathic* membranous nephropathy – no identifiable precipitating factor.

154 i. The differential diagnosis of nephrotic-range proteinuria following renal transplantation includes recurrent GN, *de novo* GN, acute allograft rejection and chronic rejection. The most common causes of recurrent GN associated with nephrotic-range proteinuria in renal transplant recipients are membranous nephropathy, FSGS and MPGN.
ii. The biopsy shows reduplication (i.e., 'splitting') of glomerular capillary basement membrane with interposition of mesangial matrix, findings characteristic of transplant glomerulopathy. Although the pathogenesis of transplant glomerulopathy is poorly understood, it is thought to be a form of chronic rejection. Patients with transplant glomerulopathy often have a progressive decline in renal function ultimately leading to allograft failure. Although the light microscopic changes of transplant glomerulopathy are similar to those seen in MPGN, there are no glomerular basement membrane deposits in transplant glomerulopathy. Thus, electron microscopy can be used to look for basement membrane deposits seen in MPGN.

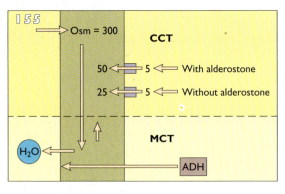

155 i. The TTKG is a tool which allows the clinician to obtain a rough idea of the processes occurring at the cortical collecting tubule (CCT), the site of potassium secretion. Under conditions of maximal aldosterone secretion, the TTKG gradient should be 8–10; under conditions in which aldosterone is suppressed (when potassium conservation is needed), it should be <5 (see **155**). The TTKG is only valid when the urine is concentrated. It presumes a urinary osmolarity of 300 mOsm/l at the CCT. Thus, if the urine osmolarity is 600 mOsm/l, 50% of the water has been removed and the final urine has twice the potassium concentration present at the CCT. The formula for TTKG is:

TTKG = (urinary K$^+$/plasma K$^+$)/(urine osmolarity/serum osmolarity)

In this patient, TTKG is (20/2.5)/(600/300) ≈ 4.
ii. This patient is appropriately conserving potassium.

Serum	Result
Sodium	138 mmol/l
Potassium	3.2 mmol/l
Chloride	108 mmol/l
Total CO_2	18 mmol/l
Creatinine	1.5 mg/dl (132 μmol/l)
Urea nitrogen	34 mg/dl (12 mmol/l)
Phosphorus	1.9 mg/dl (0.6 mmol/l)
Uric acid	2.1 mg/dl (124 μmol/l)
Serum glucose	90 mg/dl (5.0 mmol/l)

Arterial blood gas	Result
Arterial pH	7.36
Arterial pCO_2	33 mmHg

Urinalysis	Result
Urine pH	6.0
Urine glucose	3+

156 A glucagonoma was diagnosed in a 45-year-old woman who presented with weight loss, stomatitis, diabetes and necrolytic migratory erythema. Following resection of the tumour she received streptozotocin, 5-fluorouracil and dacarbazine. Prior to her fourth course of chemotherapy, the patient complained of weakness, shortness of breath and a 5 kg weight loss. Her examination was remarkable for orthostatic hypotension and her initial laboratory investigations are given (Tables).
i. What is the most likely aetiology of her low serum bicarbonate?
ii. What illnesses are associated with hypouricaemia?
iii. What is the treatment for her disorder?

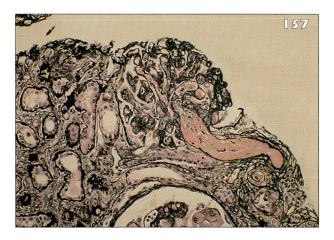

157 One week following heart transplantation, a patient develops anaemia, thrombocytopenia and acute renal failure. Immunosuppression consists of prednisone, CSA and azathioprine. A kidney biopsy was performed (**157**, courtesy of R. Hennigar, MD). What is the diagnosis?

156 i. The patient has a normal anion-gap metabolic acidosis secondary to proximal RTA (Type II). The differential diagnosis of normal anion-gap metabolic acidosis includes RTA, parenteral nutrition, gastrointestinal bicarbonate loss, ammonium chloride ingestion and partial correction of ketoacidosis.

The three types of RTA are classified according to the site involved and/or the mechanism responsible. Type I or distal RTA results from either decreased distal tubule H^+ secretion, inability to generate a negative electrochemical gradient (i.e., lumen negative) or lumen to tubule 'backleak' of excreted H^+ ions. Type II or proximal RTA results from a defect in proximal bicarbonate resorption. In addition to loss of bicarbonate there can be failure to resorb filtered uric acid, phosphorus, amino acids, potassium, glucose and sodium, resulting in hypophosphataemia, hypouricaemia, glycosuria and volume depletion (Fanconi's syndrome). Causes of Fanconi's syndrome includes tubulointerstitial diseases (Sjögren's, medullary cystic disease, renal transplantation), drugs (streptozotocin, solvent abuse, gentamicin), heavy metals (lead, mercury), secondary hyperparathyroidism with chronic hypercalcaemia and genetic diseases (Wilsons', galactosaemia, cystinosis), as well as idiopathic forms. Finally, Type IV RTA occurs when there is decreased aldosterone secretion or decreased tubular responsiveness to aldosterone.

ii. Hypouricaemia is an uncommon laboratory abnormality with a limited differential diagnosis, including medications (low-dose aspirin, probenecid, allopurinol), liver disease (decreased production), Fanconi's syndrome (increased excretion), some tumours (Hodgkin's – isolated defect in resorption), extracellular volume expansion and SIADH.

iii. Therapy includes removing the offending agent when possible (e.g., streptozotocin) and potassium phosphate and bicarbonate supplements as necessary.

157 A glomerular arteriole exhibits necrotising arteriolitis with necrosis of the smooth muscle wall ('fibrinoid necrosis') and thrombus formation, suggestive of haemolytic uraemic syndrome (HUS). In adults, HUS may occur in association with pregnancy, HIV infection, carcinomas, (especially gastric), chemotherapy with mitomycin-C or cisplatin and CSA. Endothelial injury is the present in all cases of HUS, although the aetiology remains uncertain. Abnormalities described in patients with HUS which may contribute to its pathogenesis include: (a) deficient prostacyclin synthesis by endothelial cells; (b) abnormal endothelial cell interaction with von Willebrand factor, resulting in microvasculature platelet aggregation; (c) the presence of a circulating platelet-aggregating factor.

HUS carries a more severe prognosis in adults than children, with mortality rates between 20 and 60%. HUS associated with postpartum, HIV infection and chemotherapy have the worse prognosis. Treatment involves discontinuing the offending agent (i.e., CSA), supportive treatment and plasmapheresis in severe cases.

158 This is the renal biopsy of a 28-year-old woman who was found to be diabetic at the age of 13, and has been on treatment with insulin since, though her control has always been erratic. She is now eager to become pregnant. She has a creatinine clearance of 55 ml/min and 24-hour urinary protein loss of 2.1 g. Blood pressure is

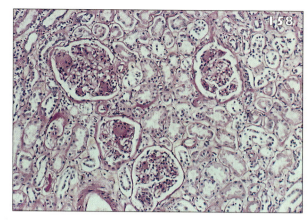

120/70 mmHg on her current treatment of lisinopril 2.5 mg daily.
i. What does the renal biopsy (**158**, courtesy of Dr A Morley) show?
ii. What advice would you give her about the possible risks of pregnancy?

159 A 45-year-old woman is referred for evaluation of renal colic and renal insufficiency. She was recently seen in the emergency department with right flank pain, radiating into the groin, which resolved after passage of a small tissue fragment identified as a necrotic papillary fragment. Her past medical history is positive for a lifelong history of tension headaches. Her medications include enalapril 5 mg daily, ranitidine 150 mg daily and an aspirin–caffeine analgesic 650 mg three to four times a day. Physical examination reveals a thin, pale woman with a blood pressure of 150/95 mmHg, and no other positive findings are elicited. Laboratory studies show serum creatinine, 3.4 mg/dl (300 μmol/l), urea nitrogen 39 mg/dl (14 mmol/l); urinalysis shows 2+ protein, 2+ blood and a specific gravity of 1.010. Her IVP is shown (**159**, courtesy of Brenda Lee Holbert). What is the most likely cause of this patient's renal failure?

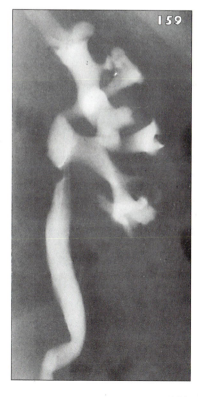

158 i. The biopsy shows the typical changes of diabetic nephropathy with glomerular nodulosclerosis.

ii. Reports of pregnancy in women with diabetic nephropathy [mostly with creatinine levels of less than 200 µmol/l (about 2.3 mg/dl) and non-nephrotic range proteinuria] suggest that proteinuria will increase during the pregnancy, to nephrotic range in 50–70% of cases, but will decline to baseline levels postpartum. Creatinine clearance may decline slightly and hypertension is likely to worsen, but these changes tend to resolve after delivery. Although most reported series are small, the evidence is that the decline in renal function is no worse than that in similar diabetic patients who have not become pregnant. Recent advances in perinatal care mean that foetal survival in diabetic nephropathy is of the order of 91%; lower than that of uncomplicated diabetes, but similar to the outcome in non-diabetic renal disease. Recent evidence suggests that improved maternal glycaemic and blood pressure control reduces the risk of spontaneous abortion, malformations, macrosomia and neonatal complications.

For this patient, improved diabetic control prior to conception is essential and close monitoring of diabetic control, blood pressure and renal function will be required throughout pregnancy. Lisinopril should be stopped (ACE inhibitors are contraindicated in pregnancy because of the risk of embryopathy and neonatal renal failure) and satisfactory blood pressure control obtained prior to conception using agents, such as methyldopa and hydralazine, which are known to be safe in pregnancy.

159 Analgesic nephropathy due to long-term consumption of aspirin is the most likely cause of her renal failure. Other analgesics (phenacetin, paracetamol and NSAIDs) alone or in combination have also been associated with this disorder. Patients with analgesic nephropathy can present with recurrent episodes of renal colic resulting from the passage of small fragments of necrotic papilla. Urinary tract obstruction can result from papillary fragments or renal calculi. Urinary tract infection is also common. The IVP shows a 'ring sign' (lower right corner) which is pathognomonic of papillary necrosis. The ring represents radiodense contrast material in the calyx surrounding a radiolucent sloughed papilla. The other calyces are also blunted and deformed.

Aspirin and paracetamol are concentrated in the renal medulla due to the countercurrent multiplying system, resulting in tubule toxicity which is exacerbated by prostaglandin inhibition, decreased medullary blood flow and ischaemia. Blood vessel damage leads to irreversible medullary ischaemia and the primary lesion of analgesic nephropathy, papillary necrosis. Tubule damage and obstruction also occur, resulting in chronic interstitial nephritis.

Patients should be instructed to cease analgesic use and be closely monitored for recidivism. Therapy is directed at preventing obstruction and infection.

160 Shown are the plain radiograph (**160a**) and MRI scan (**160b**) of a patient who, several months after a successful renal transplant, presented with hip pain on walking.
i. What abnormality is shown?
ii. What is the likely cause of this abnormality?

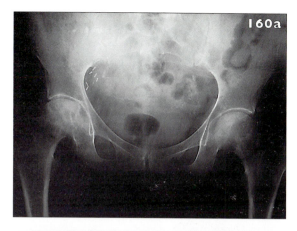

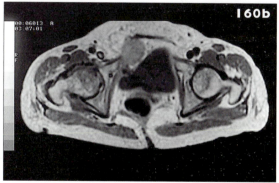

161 A 40-year-old woman with 'tubers' on her skin is admitted for abdominal and flank pain, haematuria and elevated blood pressure. Renal ultrasound shows no evidence of kidney stones or hydronephrosis, but multiple renal cysts, measuring up to 5 cm in diameter, and several echogenic, non-cystic masses are noted. By CT measurement, the density of the non-cystic masses was consistent with fat (i.e., less than water density). Unrelenting pain and haematuria finally resulted in surgical exploration; which of the following was found?
i. Renal oncocytoma.
ii. Renal angiomyolipoma (hamartoma).
iii. Renal lymphoma.
iv. Renal nephroblastoma (Wilm's tumour).

160 i. Avascular necrosis of the femoral heads is shown on both the MRI scan and the radiograph. Changes are seen earlier with MRI and this is now the imaging method of choice.
ii. In the context of renal tranplantation, avascular necrosis is most commonly seen as a complication of corticosteroid treatment and usually develops in the first year post-transplant. It most commonly affects the femoral heads and may require hip replacement.

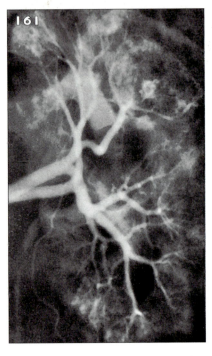

161 ii. Renal angiomyolipoma (hamartoma). Tuberous sclerosis (Bourneville's disease) is characterised by *angiomyolipomas* ('tubers') involving the face (adenoma sebaceum) and other organs, including the brain and kidneys. Angiomyolipomas are vascular masses of adipose and smooth muscle tissue, with renal involvement in 40–80% of the patients (**161**). While solitary renal angiomyolipomas have been described in patients *without* tuberous sclerosis, 80–90% of patients with bilateral renal angiomyolipomas have systemic tuberous sclerosis. The combination of cystic kidneys and angiomyolipomas is virtually pathognomonic for tuberous sclerosis. Hamartomas >4 cm in diameter may produce symptoms (e.g., flank pain, haematuria) that require partial nephrectomy or embolisation for relief. Hamartomas can also cause focal renal ischaemia, resulting in a hyperreninemic hyperaldosterone state and secondary hypertension. ESRD is unusual, although renal insufficiency may result from renal parenchymal compression by cysts and angiomyolipomas. However, the low incidence of renal failure may merely be a reflection of the high frequency of premature deaths due to central nervous system complications. Renal cell carcinoma occurs in <5% of patients with tuberous sclerosis.

Tuberous sclerosis has an autosomal dominant inheritance with a prevalence of 1:14,500, variable penetrance and a female:male ratio of 2.6:1. The genetic defect is located on chromosome 9 (TSC1) or chromosome 16 (TSC2). Interestingly, a large deletion has been described involving both TSC-2 and the adjacent PKD1 gene (the genetic defect responsible for 85% of ADPKD). Children with ADPKD and the TSC-2 gene defect develop clinical manifestations of tuberous sclerosis in early adolescence.

162 A 65-year-old man developed acute renal failure after coronary artery bypass surgery. CAVH was commenced using catheters positioned percutaneously in the left femoral artery and vein. His left foot subsequently developed the appearance shown in **162**. What is the explanation for these changes?

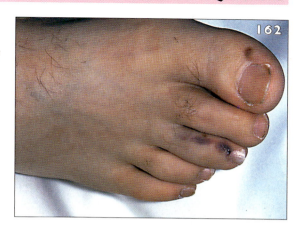

163 This CAPD patient complains of shoulder pain and stiffness.
i. What does the radiograph (**163**) show?
ii. What treatment would you recommend?

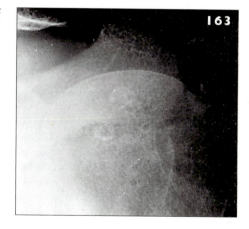

164 The iPTH (ng/l) results shown in the table were obtained during an investigative procedure in a haemodialysis patient complaining of increasing musculoskeletal pain. Six years previously he had undergone parathyroidectomy.
i. What investigative procedure has been undertaken here?
ii. What does it show?
iii. What would you do next?

Time (min)	iPTH (ng/l)
Basal	805
10	200
20	125
30	105

162 Continuous extracorporeal renal replacement therapy has become an increasingly popular treatment in intensive care units for patients with acute renal failure. Intermittent haemodialysis, even when carefully delivered, can be associated with hypotensive episodes which prolong the duration of renal failure, and can lead to undesirable swings in both fluid and uraemic toxin concentrations. Continuous therapies provide a more stable treatment, avoiding hypotension, and allowing tailored daily ultrafiltration rates to maintain fluid balance and nutritional support.

Simple extracorporeal circuits without a blood pump (CAVH, CAVHD) require both arterial and venous cannulation, typically using the femoral vessels. Arterial cannulation can be associated with complications downstream, such as lower-limb ischaemia or small peripheral vessel occlusion, due to atheromatous plaque or cholesterol embolisation (as shown here). Care should therefore be taken in using arterial catheters in any patient known to have atheromatous disease.

Concern about complications from arterial catheters has led to increased use of continuous venovenous techniques with a blood pump, using either a dual-lumen catheter or two venous catheters as vascular access (CVVH, CVVHD).

163 **i.** The radiograph shows early periarticular calcification above the left humerus. Metastatic calcification is a frequent long-term complication in both CAPD and haemodialysis patients, occurring as a result of an increased serum calcium phosphate product.
ii. The incidence of metastatic calcification in CAPD patients can be reduced by decreasing the dialysate calcium content. The use of low-calcium dialysate allows larger doses of calcium-based phosphate binders to be used to control hyperphosphataemia without these agents causing hypercalcaemia. Patients receiving vitamin D analogues to treat hyperparathyroidism may become hypercalcaemic; alteration of the dialysate calcium may allow these drugs to be tolerated without producing this effect.

164 **i.** This patient underwent a total parathyroidectomy with forearm implantation of part of one gland as an autograft. Six years later there is both biochemical and clinical evidence of recurrent hyperparathyroidism. To determine whether the autograft is responsible an ischaemic arm test has been undertaken. To do this a cannula is placed in a vein of the non-autograft arm for blood sampling. A basal sample for iPTH is taken and a tourniquet is inflated to induce ischaemia for 30 minutes; blood samples for iPTH are taken from the other arm at 10, 20 and 30 minutes. Because of its rapid half-life iPTH levels fall rapidly if the autologous forearm graft is responsible for hyperparathyroidism.
ii. The rapid fall in iPTH indicates overactivity of the forearm graft.
iii. The patient should be referred for surgical exploration of the forearm graft.

165 A peritoneal dialysis patient is admitted with peritonitis. Her past medical history is notable for a seizure disorder controlled with phenytoin. The medical house officer notifies you that the patient's phenytoin serum concentration is subtherapeutic at 7 mg/l (28 μmol/l) and suggests increasing her phenytoin dose to bring her level into the therapeutic range of 10–20 mg/l (40–80 μmol/l).
i. What action should you take?
ii. Explain why.

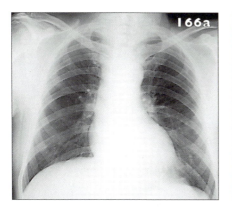 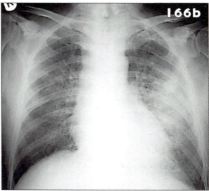

166 **166a** and **166b** are the pre- and 6-week post-operative chest radiographs of a renal transplant recipient who complained of malaise, fever, a dry cough and breathlessness. A complete blood count revealed thrombocytopenia, and liver function tests were deranged (elevated γ-GT and AST). What is the most likely diagnosis?

167 A 64-year-old patient underwent coronary artery bypass surgery 2 years following renal transplantation. During the post-operative period the patient developed a fever and this chest radiograph (**167**) was obtained. What is the differential diagnosis?

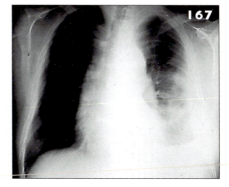

165 i. The free phenytoin level (amount of phenytoin unbound to plasma protein) should be measured. The dose of phenytoin should be adjusted only if the free phenytoin concentration is outside the therapeutic range of 1–2 mg/l (4–8 µmol/l). **ii.** The volume of distribution of many drugs may be significantly increased or decreased in renal failure. This can result from altered tissue binding, changes in protein binding or oedema. In general, plasma protein binding of acidic drugs [phenytoin, frusemide (furosemide), clofibrate] is decreased in uraemia, while basic drugs [such as quinidine or lignocaine (lidocaine)] generally have normal or only slightly decreased binding.

The free or unbound drug concentration in plasma correlates best with the concentration of the drug at its receptor. In the case of phenytoin, the free fraction of drug is 10% in patients with normal renal function. Since the normal therapeutic range for serum phenytoin is 10–20 mg/l (40–80 µmol/l), the therapeutic free phenytoin concentration would be 1–2 mg/l (4–8 µmol/l). In patients with ESRD, the free fraction of phenytoin is approximately 20%, and the total phenytoin concentration is lower due to reduced protein binding and an increased volume of distribution. Thus, the therapeutic total phenytoin concentration is typically 5–10 mg/l (20–40 µmol/l) so this patient's free concentration [20% of the total or 1.4 mg/l (5.6 µmol/l)] is actually in the therapeutic range.

The unbound drug concentration should be measured for drugs that are highly protein-bound or have a narrow therapeutic range.

166 The most likely diagnosis is CMV pneumonitis, but *Pneumocystis carinii*, bacterial infection and other viral infections should be considered. In transplant recipients the frequency and severity of CMV infection depends upon the CMV status of the donor and recipient and on the nature of the immunosuppressive regimen.

167 Pleural effusions are common after cardiothoracic surgery. However, other causes of pleural effusion should be considered, especially in an immunocompromised host. These include malignancy and infection with routine pathogens or opportunistic organisms. This patient had a tuberculous pleural effusion. In recent years tuberculosis has become increasingly common in patients with ESRD, before and after transplantation.

168 These two examples (**168a** and **168b**) of light microscopy examination of centrifuged urine come from two patients who were found to have blood in their urine on dipstick urinalysis, performed as part of routine insurance medical examinations.
i. Describe these abnormalities.
ii. What kind of underlying renal parenchymal disease is most likely to be responsible for these urinary findings?

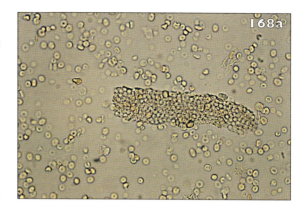

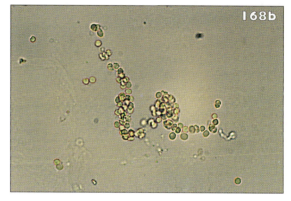

169 A 7-year-old girl presents with a history of polydipsia, polyuria, pallor, lethargy and growth retardation. Several members of her family developed ESRD prior to the age of 20 years. There is no family history of flank pain, hypertension, haematuria or nephrolithiasis. Renal ultrasound reveals small kidneys with multiple medullary cysts. She most likely has which of the following?
i. Juvenile nephronophthisis.
ii. ADPKD.
iii. Medullary sponge kidney.
iv. ARPKD.
v. Von Hippel–Lindau syndrome.

168 i. These urine specimens both show red cell casts.

ii. Red blood cell casts are diagnostic of glomerular bleeding and occur in glomeru-lonephritis. Such casts may show a wide range of different morphological appearances. The easiest to identify is the cast filled with well-defined erythrocytes, which are identical in form to those red cells which surround the cast (as in **168a**). In acid urine the erythrocytes may lose haemoglobin and remain as empty cell membranes, which are easily missed on light microscopy. The finding of a string of erythrocytes, often only one or two cells wide, without obvious surrounding protein cast matrix (as in **168b**) carries the same diagnostic implications.

The finding of red cell casts in the urine of a patient with microscopic haematuria requires further assessment of renal function, and perhaps a renal biopsy. Urological investigations, such as urine cytology, cystoscopy and IVP, are not necessary.

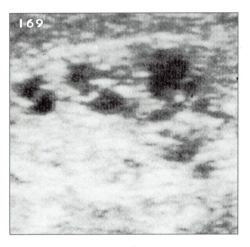

169 i. Juvenile nephronophthisis – this and medullary cystic disease are familial disorders with differing modes of inheritance, but both diseases are characterised by progressive renal failure and multiple renal cysts (1 mm to 1 cm in diameter) located in the medulla or corticomedullary junction. Renal ultrasound (**169**) or CT scan reveals normal-sized or small kidneys with smooth surfaces. Juvenile nephronophthisis is an autosomal recessive disease linked to a defect on chromosome 2 (NPH). As in our patient's kindred, ESRD typically occurs before 20 years of age, accounting for 2.4% of childhood renal failure. Renal histology reveals thin tubular basement membranes which thicken as the disease progresses, resulting in tubular atrophy, interstitial fibrosis and secondary glomerulosclerosis. Extrarenal manifestations include ocular abnormalities (retinitis pigmentosa, cataracts, amblyopia, nystagmus), cerebellar ataxia, mental retardation, bone anomalies and hepatic fibrosis.

Medullary cystic disease is an autosomal dominant disease with ESRD that develops between 20 and 50 years of age. Unlike the histological findings of juvenile nephronophthisis, thickening of tubular basement membranes does not accompany the progressive tubulointerstitial disease.

Medullary sponge kidney is typically diagnosed in the fourth or fifth decade and is characterised by dilated medullary collecting ducts and nephrolithiasis, and rarely progresses to end-stage renal failure.

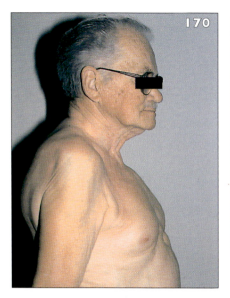

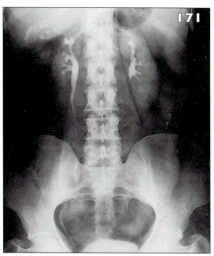

170 This patient complains that there has been a dramatic change in his body habitus since beginning maintenance immunosuppressive therapy for a kidney transplant.
i. Which medication-related effects are shown in 170?
ii. What are some of the adverse effects of corticosteroids?

171 A 19-year-old woman is prescribed a combined oestrogen–progestogen oral contraceptive containing 30 μg ethinyleostradiol. Her initial blood pressure is 124/76 mmHg but after 6 months it became 186/104 mmHg. Despite withdrawal of the medication her blood pressure remains elevated and she is referred for investigation. An IVP is undertaken (171).
i. What does the IVP show?
ii. What is the relationship between hypertension and this condition?

172 A 33-year-old man with ESRD, presumed secondary to long-standing hypertension, is referred for initiation of haemodialysis. On examination he is found to have dystrophic nails and an assortment of other skeletal abnormalities. Urinalysis reveals proteinuria and haematuria. He has a family history of renal disease, but nobody else has required dialysis or renal transplantation. Which of the following is the most likely diagnosis?
i. Alport's syndrome.
ii. Nail–patella syndrome.
iii. Hypertensive nephrosclerosis with renal osteodystrophy.
iv. Fabry's disease.
v. Von Hippel–Lindau syndrome.

170 i. This patient demonstrates classic features of Cushing's syndrome; moon facies, a buffalo hump, truncal obesity, muscle wasting and altered hair distribution. These physical changes associated with corticosteroids make it particularly difficult to enforce patient adherence to therapy, and non-adherence is a major cause of graft loss, especially among adolescents.

ii. Other adverse effects of corticosteroids include growth retardation, poor wound healing, obesity, possibly peptic ulcer disease, psychiatric disturbances, osteopenia and aseptic necrosis of bone, myopathy, hyperlipidaemia, hypertension, glucose intolerance, cataracts and acne.

171 i. The IVP shows a small right and a normal-sized left kidney. There is clubbing of the right upper pole calyces with thinning and irregularity of the overlying cortex. These appearances are characteristic of chronic pyelonephritis. The calyces can also be 'clubbed' in papillary necrosis and obstruction, but the lack of cortical scarring in the former and the presence of hydronephrosis in the latter allow differentiation.

ii. Chronic pyelonephritis is a common cause of hypertension in young women. 30% of patients have hypertension at presentation, which increases to 45% after 5 years of follow-up.

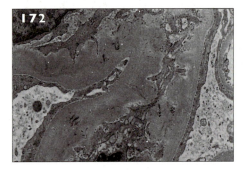

172 ii. Nail–patella syndrome (hereditary osteo-onychodysplasia), an autosomal dominant disorder linked to the genes coding for the ABO blood groups. The NPS gene coding for the α-1 chain of Type V collagen has been localised to chromosome 9. The incidence of nail–patella syndrome is 22 per million and the disease affects women and men equally. Extrarenal manifestations include nail abnormalities and deformities of the knees, elbows and iliac horns (symmetrical bony prominences of the anterior superior iliac crest). Renal involvement manifests as proteinuria, haematuria and hypertension. Of the patients, 30% progress to ESRD by age 30–50 years. Renal histology reveals a mottled or 'moth-eaten' appearance of the GBM on electron microscopy (as in **172**). Intramembranous lesions are composed of abnormally distributed Type III and IV collagen fibrils. Renal transplantation has been successful without recurrence of the GBM lesions.

173 A 4-year-old boy presents with severe left flank pain. An IVP revealed left-sided hydronephrosis and obstruction of the ureteropelvic junction. An ultrasound examination was then performed (173).
i. What is the differential diagnosis?
ii. What does the ultrasound show?

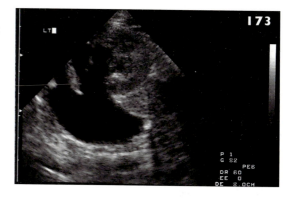

174 Shown (174) is the urine microscopy from a 5-year-old child who presented with oliguria, haematuria and signs of volume overload (oedema, hypertension, raised JVP) 2 weeks after an attack of tonsillitis.
i. What is the diagnosis?
ii. What is the most likely cause?

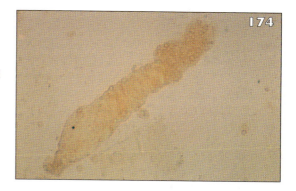

175 A 56-year-old man with long-standing peripheral vascular disease presents with increasing dyspnoea. On examination there was peripheral oedema and the jugular venous pressure was elevated. Plasma creatinine was 2 mg/dl (170 µmol/l). Cardiac echo showed normal left ventricular function. After an initial imaging procedure, renal angiography was undertaken (175).
i. What abnormalities are seen?
ii. What are the therapeutic options?

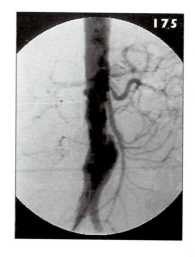

173 i. The differential diagnosis includes partial ureteropelvic junction obstruction or an obstructing renal calculus.

ii. The renal ultrasound showed left-sided hydronephrosis and a radiolucent calculus at the ureteropelvic junction, which was not visible on IVP. Since the stone is approximately 3 mm in diameter, it is likely that the child will pass the stone spontaneously. Therefore, conservative therapy with intravenous fluids and analgesics is the appropriate initial treatment.

Biochemical factors	Acute nephritic syndrome	Nephrotic syndrome
Oedema	++	+++
Blood pressure	Raised	Normal or raised
JVP	Raised	Normal or low
Proteinuria	+/++	++++
Haematuria	+++	+/–
Serum albumin	Normal	Low

174 i. The clinical presentation is acute nephritic syndrome. It is distinct from nephrotic syndrome in its characteristic form (Table), but many patients with GN present with some features of both, so-called 'nephritic–nephrotic' syndrome.

ii. This is likely to be post-streptococcal GN, which would be supported by serological evidence of recent streptococcal infection (raised antistreptolysin 'O' titre) and a low serum C3. An identical pattern of renal disease may follow infection with many organisms other than the streptococci.

175 i. The angiogram was performed after an ultrasound had shown a small (7 cm) right and a normal-sized left kidney. The angiogram shows the catheter in the right common iliac artery. There is an aneurysm of the lower aorta; the right renal artery is completely occluded and there is a stenosis just beyond the origin of the left renal artery.

ii. Angioplasty should be considered and if the stenosis recurs rapidly, then an intra-arterial stent could be inserted. If stenting is not possible, then surgery might be considered.

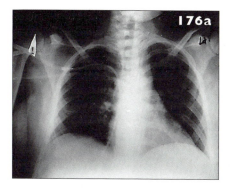 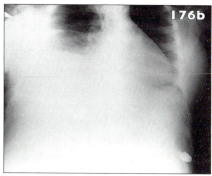

176 A 17-year-old woman presented with acute renal transplant rejection. A single lumen haemodialysis catheter was positioned via the right subclavian vein. A chest radiograph (**176a**) showed the catheter tip extending beyond the cardiac silhouette. Shortly after repositioning the catheter over a guide wire, the patient collapsed with dyspnoea, chest discomfort and hypotensive shock. A repeat radiograph (**176b**) was taken shortly before the patient died. Explain the nature of this fatal complication of subclavian cannulation for haemodialysis vascular access.

177 A 21-year-old woman with RA is referred for evaluation of proteinuria. She has no other health problems. Her RA was originally treated with aspirin, NSAIDs and low-dose glucocorticoids. Although her symptoms improved she continued to have progression of her disease. Therapy with once weekly intramuscular gold–sodium thiomalate 50 mg was initiated 6 months ago. At her previous clinic visit, the patient was

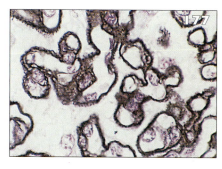

found to have 2+ proteinuria and 1+ blood on urinalysis. Other laboratory analyses are normal, except for a serum albumin of 25 g/l and serum cholesterol of 250 mg/dl (6.5 mmol/l). A 24-hour urine collection reveals 6.1 g protein/day. A renal biopsy was performed and is shown (**177**, methenamine silver trichrome stain of a representative section of one glomerulus, courtesy of Sheldon I. Bastacky). What is the differential diagnosis of the nephrotic syndrome in this patient?

176 The patient was asymptomatic during and following the initial catheter insertion, and the radiograph was reported as showing the tip of the catheter beyond the cardiac silhouette, probably within a hepatic vein. Subsequent post-mortem examination showed that during the repositioning of the catheter the tip perforated the right atrium, penetrating the visceral and parietal pericardium and entering the right pleural space. Death was caused by massive haemorrhage into the right haemothorax.

Haemothorax can occur as a consequence of laceration of the wall of the subclavian vein, inadvertent puncture of the subclavian artery during the insertion procedure or from the infusion of transfused blood through a misplaced catheter. However, life-threatening haemothorax due to a haemodialysis catheter is usually a consequence of vascular perforation. Puncture of the superior vena cava or right atrium may occur during the insertion procedure. The risk can be reduced by the use of catheters made from plastic that softens at body temperature. A catheter that has become partially extruded should never by blindly pushed back in.

177 The causes of proteinuria in this patient include drug toxicity from gold or NSAIDs or a primary glomerular disorder. Transient proteinuria, nephrotic syndrome and microscopic haematuria are well-described complications of gold therapy and tend to be more common with higher doses. The incidence of proteinuria is variable, occurring in 0–26% of patients receiving this drug. Nephrotic syndrome is less frequent, about 3% in one study of 75 patients. In patients with nephrotic syndrome, the most common lesion seen on renal biopsy is membranous glomerulopathy. **177** demonstrates the characteristic subepithelial 'spikes' along glomerular basement membrane. A unique morphological finding in patients with gold-induced nephrosis (in contrast to idiopathic membranous GN) is the demonstration on electron microscopy of gold inclusions in the mesangium, glomerular epithelial cells and proximal convoluted tubules.

Rarely, NSAIDs have also been associated with nephrotic syndrome. Histologically, minimal change disease (MCD) is most common, although, in contrast to idiopathic MCD, a superimposed mononuclear cell interstitial infiltrate is usually present with NSAID-induced nephrosis. Proteinuria has also been reported in patients receiving penicillamine for RA. When nephrotic syndrome complicates therapy with penicillamine, the histological lesion is usually membranous GN. Typically, proteinuria resolves slowly after gold or penicillamine therapy is withdrawn. Primary glomerular disorders to consider also in this patient include secondary amyloidosis or one of the idiopathic nephrotic syndromes.

178 A 13-year old girl is admitted with generalised echymoses, following a diarrhoeal illness. She is afebrile and mildly hypertensive. Laboratory values reveal anaemia, thrombocytopenia, hyperbilirubinaemia and azotaemia [BUN 88 mg/dl (31 mmol/l), serum creatinine 7 mg/dl (620 µmol/l)]. PT and PTT are normal, and blood cultures are negative. A peripheral blood smear is shown (178, courtesy of V. Silva, MD).
i. What is the most likely diagnosis?
ii. What therapy is indicated?

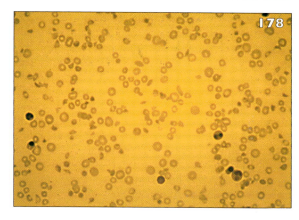

179 This skull radiograph (179) is from a 50-year-old man who was referred with hypertension. He also complained of a persistent headache and glycosuria was noted on urinalysis.
i. What abnormalities are seen on the radiograph (179)?
ii. What other features in the history and examination could help in making the diagnosis?
iii. What investigations would you undertake?
iv. What is the relationship between the hypertension and the underlying diagnosis?

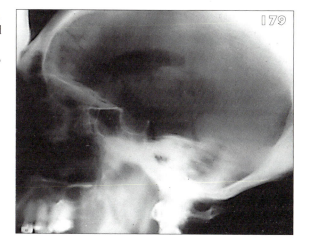

178 i. The peripheral smear shows schistocytes, fragmented and nucleated RBCs, suggestive of a microvascular haemolytic process. The combination of microangiopathic haemolytic anaemia, thrombocytopenia and acute renal failure suggests HUS. Disseminated intravascular coagulation (DIC), malignant hypertension and systemic vasculitis should be considered in the differential diagnosis. HUS is characterised by the formation of platelet thrombi in the renal microcirculation, resulting from endothelial cell injury. Haemolysis results from mechanical fragmentation of RBCs. In children, 90% of cases present in an epidemic form, associated with prodromal diarrhoea and evidence of infection with verotoxin-producing *E. coli* (VTEC, serotype O157:H7) or *Shigella* organisms. A sporadic form of HUS is the most common presentation in adults; it is not associated with diarrhoea or VTEC infection. The prognosis differs between the two presentations. Acute renal failure requiring dialysis occurs in more than 50% of patients with epidemic HUS, but the prognosis for renal recovery is good and mortality is less than 10%. The sporadic form of HUS has a grim prognosis: mortality is 25% and end-stage renal failure may develop in 25% of survivors.

ii. Supportive care is indicated in milder cases of epidemic HUS. Plasma exchange is usually recommended for patients with severe anaemia, or renal failure requiring dialysis. To avoid the risk of volume overload plasma exchange is preferred to plasma infusion and is performed daily until improvement in the microangiopathic anaemia and other clinical parameters are seen. Antibiotics, which eradicate enteric pathogens, do not alter the course of the disease. Neither heparin nor thrombolytics are useful; moreover, they may cause severe bleeding and should be avoided. Corticosteroids and cytotoxic agents are usually reserved for recurrent cases, although their benefit remains unproved. Prostacyclin and vitamin E, an antioxidant agent, have been reported to be of benefit in uncontrolled studies.

179 i. There is enlargement of the sella turcica and frontal sinuses consistent with acromegaly.

ii. Other symptoms and signs of acromegaly include increasing shoe size, changes in facial appearance, enlargement of the hands and a visual field defect (bitemporal hemianopia).

iii. The definitive investigation for the diagnosis of acromegaly is the measurement of growth hormone during a glucose tolerance test – normally growth hormone concentration is suppressed. Measurement of serum IGF-1 can be used as a screening test.

iv. It is reported that up to 45% of patients with acromegaly have hypertension. Predisposing factors include sodium retention and increased renin levels.

180 A renal transplant recipient presented with worsening hypertension and a loud systolic bruit was heard over the allograft. He had received a mis-matched cadaveric renal transplant 12 months previously, which was complicated by a single episode of biopsy-proven acute rejection. How is the finding on the arteriogram (**180**) related?

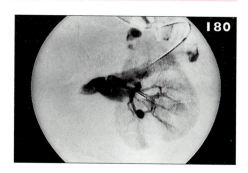

181 A 35-year-old man with three episodes of nephrolithiasis is referred for evaluation. Analysis of one of his stones reveals that it is composed of calcium oxalate with a uric acid core. He follows no specific diet and takes no medications. No family members have nephrolithiasis. His physical examination is normal and the results of two random 24-hour urine tests while eating his usual diet are given (Table).

Test	Random	Random	Units
Volume	1200	1100	ml
pH	5.5	5.5	–
Calcium	180	170	mg/day
Uric acid	850	900	mg/day
Creatinine	1500	1450	mg/day
Urea nitrogen	11300	11000	mg/day
Sodium	170	150	mmol/day
Magnesium	7	8	mmol/day
Oxalate	23	19	mg/day
Citrate	350	450	mg/day

i. What metabolic abnormality is responsible for his nephrolithiasis?
ii. What therapy would you prescribe?

182 i. What is shown in **182**?
ii. What systemic complication can this structure cause?

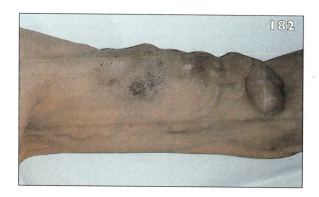

180 The arteriogram demonstrates an arteriovenous fistula in the lower pole of the kidney associated with a wedge-shaped cortical perfusion defect. Such complications of renal biopsies are unusual, but have been reported to cause secondary hypertension. The mechanism has been attributed to localised renal ischaemia and consequent increased renin production. In the occasional case where blood pressure control has been refractory to antihypertensive medications (e.g., ACE inhibitors), selective vascular ablation has been successful.

181 i. Low urine volume and hyperuricosuria are potential factors contributing to his nephrolithiasis. Hyperuricosuria is a risk factor for uric acid stones, but uric acid can also serve as a nidus for calcium oxalate stone formation. In addition, the solubility of urate is decreased in an acidic urine.

ii. Therapy includes (a) encouraging enough fluid intake to achieve a urine output >2 l/day (because of insensible fluid losses the patient is likely need to drink ≥ 3 l of fluid per day), (b) modest protein restriction (about 1 g/kg/day) to reduce urine acidity and to decrease purine intake, and (c) allopurinol to inhibit uric acid production and to decrease uric acid excretion. It is important to repeat the urine collections 4–8 weeks after initiation of therapy to confirm that therapy was successful.

182 i. This is an arteriovenous fistula (AVF) used for chronic haemodialysis vascular access. A native AVF is created typically by an end-to-side venous-to-arterial anastomosis using a nearby vein and either the radial artery at the wrist or the brachial artery at the antecubital fossa (as shown here). Transmission of arterial blood pressure results in 'arterialisation' of the venous segment of the AVF, which becomes dilated and amenable to haemodialysis needle puncture after a post-operative maturation period of about 6–8 weeks. The AVF, initially described by Brescia and Cimino, remains the 'gold standard' vascular access because of good long-term patency and low rates of infection or thrombosis.

ii. An AVF may be associated with a number of local complications, such as poor flow, thrombosis, infection, aneurysmal dilatation, distal extremity ischaemia and oedema of the hand. In patients with severe cardiac dysfunction, AVF creation may be associated with significant cardiovascular decompensation leading to high output congestive cardiac failure. Cardiac failure is very unusual with radiocephalic fistulae, but is more common in patients with either an upper arm AVF or multiple fistulae. Doppler studies suggest that mature native fistulae have mean blood flow rates of around 800 ml/min. Cardiac failure is likely to develop if fistula flow exceeds 20% of the cardiac output.

183 An 80-year-old woman is admitted with acute diverticular disease. She is febrile and blood cultures show a significant growth of *E. coli* which is resistant to all agents except gentamicin. Her plasma creatinine is 1.1 mg/dl (100 µmol/l) and she is treated with gentamicin 1 mg/kg i.v. three times a day. Over the next 4 days her plasma creatinine rises to 300 µmol/l (3.4 mg/dl). A renal biopsy is obtained (183).

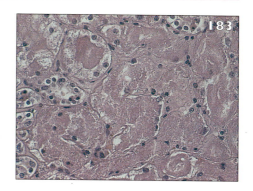

i. What does the renal biopsy show?
ii. What is the cause of the renal impairment?

184 What explanations may there be for the biochemical changes (Table) in this patient?

Biochemical factors	At admission	One week later
Serum urea nitrogen	17.4 mg/dl (6.2 mmol/l)	102 mg/dl (36.4 mmol/l)
Serum creatinine	1.1 mg/dl (103 µmol/l)	2.6 mg/dl (234 µmol/l)
Serum sodium	140 mmol/l	132 mmol/l
Serum potassium	4.2 mmol/l	3.2 mmol/l
Serum albumin	18 g/l	22 g/l
Urine protein	12.6 g/24 h	11.4 g/24 h

185 A 42-year-old woman with lymphoma develops acute renal failure 48 hours following her first course of chemotherapy. There has been no hypotension. Her examination shows generalised wasting, cervical lymphadeno-pathy, splenomegaly, hepatomegaly and no oedema. Urine output was 300 ml/day and her serum laboratory studies revealed creatinine 5.2 mg/dl (460 mmol/l), urea nitrogen 80 mg/dl (29 µmol/l), potassium

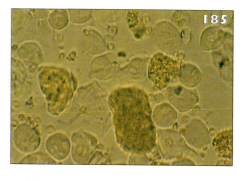

5.2 mmol/l, bicarbonate 18 mmol/l, uric acid 19 mg/dl (1130 µmol/l), phosphorus 13.2 mg/dl (4.3 mmol/l) and total calcium 6.0 mg/dl (1.5 mmol/l). Her fractional excretion of sodium was 3% and her urinalysis is shown in 185.
i. What was the cause of her acute renal failure?
ii. What therapy should be instituted?

183 i. The renal biopsy shows acute tubular necrosis and a mild interstitial infiltrate.
ii. The ATN was caused by gentamicin. In the elderly, renal function is often impaired despite a 'normal' serum creatinine. Dehydration, hypokalaemia, hyponatraemia and acidosis also predispose to the development of gentamicin nephrotoxicity.

184 (a) *Volume contraction.* Patients with nephrotic syndrome are commonly volume-contracted because of reduced colloid oncotic pressure due to hypoalbuminaemia. Pre-renal azotaemia may therefore develop spontaneously, particularly if there is very heavy proteinuria.

More commonly, volume contraction is provoked by *diuretics*, especially if there is a rapid diuresis. This is more likely in this case given the concomitant fall in serum sodium and potassium concentrations and the disproportionate rise in urea compared to creatinine.
(b) *Renal vein thrombosis.* The sudden decline in renal function may also be explained by the development of renal vein thrombosis, a complication provoked by both volume contraction and altered patterns of circulating coagulation proteins to a procoagulant profile – typically raised fibrinogen and factors V, VII and X (increased hepatic synthesis) and lowered antithrombin III (increased urinary loss).
(c) *Catabolic effect of corticosteroids.* The disproportionate rise in urea may also indicate the catabolic response to high-dose corticosteroids. Hypokalaemia may also follow corticosteroid therapy.
(d) *Progression of the underlying glomerulonephritis.* There may be a rapidly progressive glomerular disease underlying the initial presentation of nephrotic syndrome. This would be suggested by an active urine sediment (red cells and red cell casts as well as proteinuria), but can only be confirmed by renal biopsy.
(e) *Acute renal failure.* This is an occasional complication of minimal change nephrotic syndrome, even in the absence of any of the explanations given above. It is not well understood, but severe intrarenal oedema, which impairs blood flow and tubular function by a mechanical effect, has been proposed. Renal function improves spontaneously with diuresis.

185 i. Her urinalysis shows red blood cells, renal tubular epithelial cells and a muddy brown granular cast. The history, serum chemistries and urine findings are compatible with acute uric acid nephropathy secondary to tumour lysis syndrome. Acute uric acid nephropathy causes acute renal failure due to precipitation of uric acid within tubules, resulting from increased uric acid production following massive cell necrosis, as can be seen following chemotherapy. Acute uric acid nephropathy is often associated with hyperkalaemia, hyperphosphataemia and hypocalcaemia.
ii. The most important therapy is prevention. These measures include hydration, urine alkalinisation and pretreatment with allopurinol. Once acute renal failure develops patients may require dialysis.

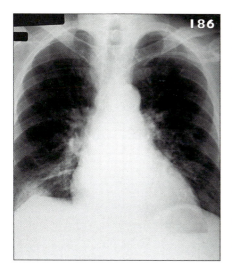

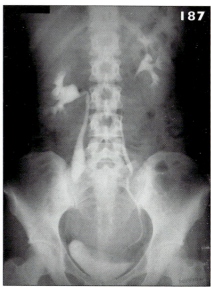

186 This patient was doing well 5 years after transplantation when he developed fever, chills, headache and a stiff neck. This chest radiograph (**186**) was obtained.
i. What is the differential diagnosis in this patient?
ii. What diagnostic tests should be performed next?

187 What does this IVP (**187**) show?

188 Shown (**188**) are serial plasma urea, creatinine and serum albumin levels in a group of patients followed over 3 years of CAPD treatment.
i. How would you determine whether these patients were adequately dialysed over this period?
ii. Why do the urea and creatinine levels rise over the first 2 years in these patients?

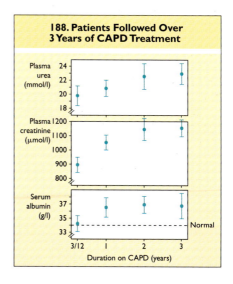

153

186 i. The constellation of fever, headache and stiff neck suggests meningitis and/or encephalitis. A number of common pathogens and opportunistic organisms can cause central nervous system infections in renal transplant recipients. Meningitis may be caused by common pathogens, such as *Haemophilus influenza*, *Neisseria meningitidis* and *Streptococcus pneumoniae*, or by opportunistic organisms, such as *Cryptococcus neoformans*, *Listeria monocytogenes*, *Mycobacterium tuberculosis*, *Coccidioides immitis*, *Histoplasma capsulatum* and *Candida albicans*. Focal brain abscesses may be caused by common Gram-positive and Gram-negative bacterial pathogens or by opportunistic organisms, such as *Aspergillus fumigatus*, *Nocardia asteroides* and *Toxoplasma gondii*. This patient had cryptococcal meningitis with pulmonary involvement.

ii. Generally, a CT or MRI of the brain should be performed first. If there is no intracerebral mass, a lumbar puncture should be obtained. Cerebral spinal fluid should be sent for Gram, Ziehl–Neelsen and India ink stains, as well as for cell count, chemistries and cultures. A test for cryptococcal antigen should also be peformed.

187 The IVP shows dilatation of the right pelvicalyceal system and the right ureter to the level of the pelvic brim. An involuting, but still enlarged, uterus is also visible on this early postpartum film.

Dilatation of the pelvicalyceal systems and ureters occurs in the first trimester and persists until the early postpartum, usually returning to normal within 15 weeks of delivery. The dilatation is usually greater on the right and stops at the level of the pelvic brim. Hormonal factors, inefficient peristalsis and obstruction caused by the enlarging uterus (plus dilated ovarian venous plexus, uterine veins or iliac vessels) are all postulated causes of the dilatation. In this film there is compression of the right ureter by the ovarian vein.

188 i. Assessing the adequacy of peritoneal dialysis is difficult. In the clinical evaluation of the patient it is important to establish whether uraemic symptoms, fluid balance and nutritional status improve after starting dialysis and whether this improvement is maintained. Changes in plasma urea and creatinine are not useful measures of peritoneal dialysis adequacy and hypoalbuminaemia often occurs at a late stage. Measurement of urea and creatinine clearance from 24-hour urine and effluent collections may provide a guide to dialysis adequacy. In practice it is most important to identify those patients with loss of residual renal function as they are at most risk of inadequate dialysis.

ii. The rise in plasma urea and creatinine concentrations probably reflects loss of residual renal function. Changes in plasma urea and creatinine levels may be misleading, since they are also influenced by protein intake (urea) and changes in lean body mass (creatinine).

189 A 10-year-old boy presents with a history of recurrent haematuria. Multiple urological examinations (cystogram and retrograde pyelograms) reveal no evidence of genitourinary structural abnormalities. The family has a history of renal failure, ocular abnormalities and deafness. A renal biposy is undertaken and the EM is shown in **189**. Which of the following is the most likely diagnosis?

i. IgA nephropathy.
ii. Thin basement membrane disease.
iii. Alport's syndrome.
iv. Juvenile nephronophthisis.

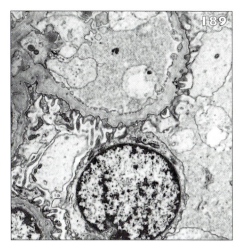

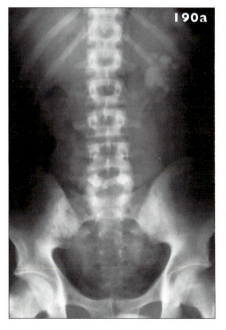

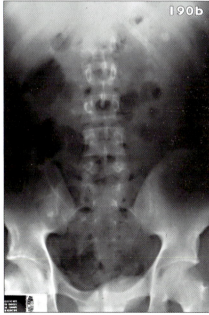

190 The two plain abdominal radiographs shown are before (**190a**) and after (**190b**) a medical treatment (no surgery).

i. What abnormality is shown?
ii. What is the likely cause and what was the medical treatment?

189 iii. Alport's syndrome (hereditary nephritis) is an X-linked disorder featuring progressive glomerular disease, and ocular and auditory abnormalities. Female carriers may develop haematuria, but do not develop progressive renal failure. The exception is the rare occurrence of autosomal recessive forms of hereditary nephritis, where the clinical presentation in both women and men is identical. In 15% of Alport's cases there is no family history, suggesting the spontaneous appearance of a new mutation.

Typically patients present in childhood with asymptomatic haematuria and/or proteinuria. Progressive renal disease leads to end-stage renal failure which has a bimodal age distribution (early onset between 16 and 35 years or delayed onset at 45 to 60 years old). Sensorineural hearing loss (30–50%), ocular anomalies (spherophakia, myopia, retinitis pigmentosa, anterior lenticonus, cataracts, perimacular retinal lesions) and megathrombocytopenia may also be seen in some kindreds with Alport's syndrome. Renal biopsy initially reveals thinning of the glomerular basement membranes, but as the disease progresses the basement membranes become thickened and lammelated. The electron microscopy from this patient shows the characteristic longitudinal splitting of the basement membrane.

The diverse manifestations of hereditary nephritis suggest a defect in connective tissue structure. Indeed, a number of genetic mutations or deletions involving the α-5 chain of type IV collagen, which is located on the X chromosome, have been described in different kindreds with Alport's syndrome. In addition, defects in the genes encoding the α-3 and α-4 chains on chromosome 2 have been described in some families. The α-3, α-4 and α-5 chains combine to form the collagen network of the glomerular basement membrane.

190 i. The radiograph before treatment (**190a**) shows a staghorn calculus on the left. **ii.** The most likely cause is a cystine stone that has been treated with increasing fluid intake, alkalinisation and oral penicillamine. Cystine stones are responsible for 1–2% of all urinary calculi. They are caused by the condition cystinuria, an autosomal recessive (complete and incomplete) transport defect of the amino acids cystine, lysine, ornithine and arginine causing excessive excretion of cystine. The solubility of cystine is usually 1–2 mmol/l (250–500 mg/l) and excretion in affected individuals is usually between 2–15 mmol/24 h (250–3600 mg/24 h), so the fluid intake necessary to keep cystine soluble can be calculated. Alkalinisation also increases the solubility of cystine. Penicillamine is reserved for those cases unresponsive to the above therapy because it causes side effects in a majority of patients, including rashes, abnormalities of sense and smell, a serum sickness-type picture and drug-induced SLE. Because the only calculi that can dissolve with medical treatment are uric acid and cystine, and since uric acid calculi are radiolucent, this patient most likely had a cystine calculus.

191 A 35-year-old white man who recently received a cadaveric renal transplant is seen in transplant clinic. His post-operative course was uncomplicated and his medications include CSA, azathioprine, prednisone and sulfamethoxazole-trimethoprim. Serum laboratory values are: Na^+ 140 mmol/l, K^+ 6.8 mmol/l, Cl^- 100 mmol/l, HCO_3^- 24 mmol/l, creatinine 1.5 mg/dl (133 μmol/l) and BUN 15 mg/dl (5.4 mmol/l). ECG reveals peaked T waves and a prolonged P-R interval.

i. Initial therapy should include:
(a) Intravenous insulin with glucose.
(b) Intravenous calcium gluconate.
(c) Inhaled beta₂ agonist.
(d) Intravenous bicarbonate.
(e) Cation-exchange resin.
(f) Diuretics.

ii. Likely contributing factors to his hyperkalaemia include:
(a) CSA.
(b) Sulphamethoxazole.
(c) Trimethoprim.
(d) Azathioprine.
(e) Renal insufficiency.

192 A 23-year-old Africo-American man with sickle-cell anaemia was admitted to hospital in pain crisis. The patient's history is notable only for his sickle-cell disease. Physical examination shows the patient to be hypertensive (180/110 mmHg) and in acute distress secondary to pain.

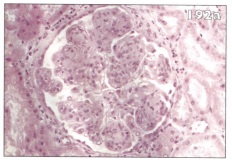

Urinalysis reveals haematuria and proteinuria; oval fat bodies and granular casts are also seen. A 24-hour urine collection reveals a creatinine clearance of 35 ml/min and a protein excretion of 6.2 g/day. Further serological and laboratory workups are negative. Following resolution of the patient's sickle crisis a renal biopsy is performed. Two representative glomeruli are shown in **192a** (H&E stain, courtesy of Sheldon I. Bastacky) and **192b** (methenamine silver trichrome stain, courtesy of Sheldon I. Bastacky).

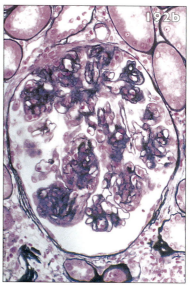

i. What glomerular lesion is present?
ii. Is this glomerular lesion related to the patient's sickle-cell disease?
iii. What other abnormalities can be seen in this condition?

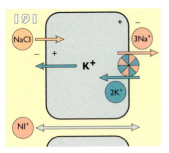

191 i. This patient has hyperkalaemia with adverse effects on the cardiac conduction system. Initial therapy should be to stabilise the myocardial membrane by driving potassium from the extracellular to the intracellular space. Calcium salts increase the threshold potential of the myocardium and insulin is thought to lower the serum potassium by increasing the transmembrane shift of potassium by activating Na^+/K^+-ATP-ase. Similarly, beta$_2$ agonists drive potassium into cells. These work best with haemodialysis patients and probably should only be used as adjuvant therapy with insulin and glucose. The effect of bicarbonate is unpredictable and should not be relied upon as sole therapy. Hyperkalaemia should also be treated with oral cation-exchange resins and by increasing potassium excretion with loop diuretics.

ii. Urinary potassium excretion is almost entirely by secretion of potassium by the principal cell of the CCT (see 191). The reabsorption of sodium by the CCT sodium channels and its relative impermeability to chloride creates an electrochemical gradient favouring movement of potassium from the tubule to the lumen. In addition, the reabsorption of sodium activates the basolateral Na^+/K^+-ATP-ase which drives potassium from the blood to the tubule cell. Then, potassium is secreted into the tubule lumen as a function of its concentration and electrochemical gradient. The principal hormone regulating this process is aldosterone, which activates the Na^+/K^+-ATP-ase and increases the number and activity of the sodium channels. Trimethoprim causes hyperkalaemia by inhibiting sodium channels. CSA is commonly associated with hyperkalaemia, but the mechanism is not entirely clear. Sulfamethoxazole does not cause hyperkalaemia. Generally, this degree of renal impairment would not be associated with hyperkalaemia.

192 i. The lobulated appearance of the glomerular tuft in 192a is consistent with MPGN (MCGN). The glomerulus in 192b has been stained with methenamine silver trichrome to accentuate the basement membranes. Duplication of these membranes is evident in several of the glomerular capillary loops, consistent with MPGN.

ii. Yes, sickle-cell anaemia is one of the secondary causes of MPGN and occurs in approximately 4% of patients with haemoglobin SS. Patients typically present with renal insufficiency early in their third decade. Progressive renal damage is associated with hypertension, microscopic haematuria, proteinuria and nephrotic syndrome. These patients are at greater risk of premature death, with about 50% dying within 4 years of the diagnosis of renal failure.

iii. Impaired urinary concentrating ability is one of the first renal disturbances seen in patients with sickle cell anaemia. Sickling of the blood impairs renal blood flow to the medulla and prevents the maintenance of medullary hypertonicity necessary for maximal concentration. Long-standing sickling leads to ischaemia, followed by papillary necrosis. These patients may also develop a hyperkalaemic, distal RTA.

193 In May 1995 an elderly diabetic with nephropathy complains of profuse diarrhoea and weakness. Since January 1994 he has been taking a converting enzyme inhibitor and a diuretic. His blood pressure is 118/60 mmHg, serum electrolytes are normal, but the serum creatinine is 3.8 mg/dl (336 µmol/l). A review of his records is given (Table).
i. Is his course compatible with progressive diabetic nephropathy?
ii. What are the diagnostic possibilities?
iii. Are converting enzyme inhibitors contraindicated in this patient?

Test	Jan 1991	Jan 1992	Jan 1993	Jan 1994	Jan 1995
Blood pressure (mmHg)	132/88	128/86	134/88	136/88	138/86
Serum creatinine (mg/dl)	1.1	1.3	1.5	1.8	2.2
(µmol/l)	97	115	133	160	194

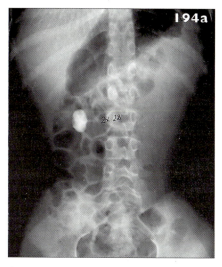
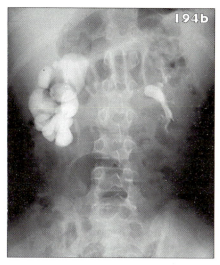

194 A 7-year-old boy presents with severe right flank pain. The plain abdominal film (**194a**) and IVP (**194b**) are shown.
i. What is the abnormality present on the radiograph?
ii. What is the appropriate management?

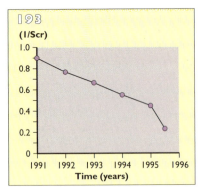

193 i. In most patients with chronic renal failure, the GFR declines at a constant rate and hence the slope of GFR vs time is linear. Since the rate of decline in renal function is predictable, deviations from linearity can be used to detect a superimposed condition. Clinically, GFR is estimated from the creatinine clearance, whereby (Scr = serum creatinine):

creatinine clearance = urine creatinine/Scr

Since creatinine excretion is relatively constant, this equation can be expressed as:

creatinine clearance = k x (1/Scr)

Thus, plotting (1/Scr) vs time is equivalent to plotting creatinine clearance (GFR) vs time.

The plot of (1/Scr) vs time here (193) indicates that renal function declined at a constant rate between January 1991 and January 1995. However, the (1/Scr) value from May 1995 does not fall on the line predicted from the previous serum creatinine values, suggesting an acute deterioration of renal function not related to the progression of the underlying disease.

ii. Acute renal failure secondary to volume depletion from diarrhoea is the most likely diagnosis. In sodium-depleted states, the maintenance of GFR is dependent on angiotensin II-mediated efferent arteriolar vasoconstriction. When volume depletion occurs in a patient in whom angiotensin II formation is inhibited (i.e., taking converting enzyme inhibitors), renal failure can occur. The differential diagnosis should also include obstructive nephropathy secondary to a neurogenic bladder, renal arterial occlusive disease, use of NSAIDs and papillary necrosis.

iii. Acutely, converting enzyme inhibitors should be discontinued. After volume repletion, converting enzyme inhibitors can usually be resumed safely, since GFR is no longer dependent upon angiotensin II.

194 i. The plain abdominal film (194a) shows a 2 cm opaque right renal calculi, which is seen to be obstructing the ureteropelvic junction on the IVP (194b). A renal calculi of this size will not pass spontaneously.

ii. Extracorporeal shock wave lithotripsy (ESWL) has provided an alternative to surgery in many cases. Under anaesthesia, the stone is manipulated into the renal pelvis using a ureteral catheter and then a ureteral stent is placed at the site of obstruction. The stone is then subjected to ESWL and the fragments allowed to pass spontaneously. Stone fragments are sent for analysis and a metabolic evaluation is then performed to determine the appropriate therapy for the nephrolithiasis.

195 A 25-year-old man with Alport's syndrome progresses to end-stage renal failure and is started on haemodialysis. Several years later, he receives a cadaveric renal transplant and is maintained on oral prednisone, CSA and azathioprine. This patient is at increased risk for developing which of the following in his transplanted kidney?
i. Recurrent Alport's disease.
ii. Anti-GBM (glomerular basement membrane) antibody disease.
iii. Corticosteroid-induced diabetic nephropathy.
iv. Juvenile nephronophthisis.
v. CSA nephrotoxicity.

196 A 78-year-old white woman presents to her physician complaining of weakness. She is in good health except for mild hypertension controlled with hydrochlorothiazide 25 mg p.o. q day. She stated that her appetite has decreased and that her diet consists primarily of juices, tea and cereals. Physical examination was unremarkable with normal blood pressure and no oedema. Significant laboratory values are given (Table).

i. The most likely cause of this patient's hyponatraemia is:
(a) SIADH.
(b) Psychogenic polydipsia.
(c) Thiazide diuretic.
(d) Salt-losing nephropathy.
ii. Appropriate treatment options include:
(a) Fluid restriction.
(b) Discontinuing thiazide diuretic.
(c) Normal saline.
(d) Hypertonic saline.

Serum	Value	Urine	Value
Na^+	119 mmol/l	Osmolarity	310 mOsm/l
K^+	3.1 mmol/l	Na^+	30 mmol/l
Cl^-	82 mmol/l	Cl^-	52 mmol/l
HCO_3^-	25 mmol/l	K^+	20 mmol/l
BUN	9 mg/dl (3.2 mmol/l)		
Creatinine	1.0 mg/dl (90 μmol/l)		
Uric acid	6.8 mg/dl (400 μmol/l)		

195 ii. Anti-GBM antibody disease – some patients with Alport's syndrome form anti-GBM antibodies following renal transplantation. The risk appears to be greatest in those with a large deletion in the gene coding for the α-3 chain of type IV collagen, in which case the Goodpasture antigen is not expressed. The Goodpasture antigen in the renal graft is recognised as foreign since it was not expressed in the Alport patients' native kidneys. Glomerular deposition of anti-GBM antibodies is associated with Goodpasture's disease in about 5% of patients with Alport's syndrome, usually manifesting within the first year following transplantation. Since this incidence is low, transplantation is not contraindicated in patients with hereditary nephritis.

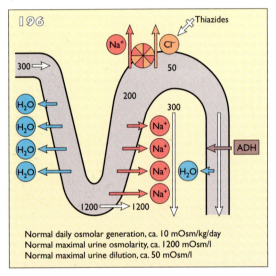

Normal daily osmolar generation, ca. 10 mOsm/kg/day
Normal maximal urine osmolarity, ca. 1200 mOsm/l
Normal maximal urine dilution, ca. 50 mOsm/l

196 i. (c) The most likely reason for this woman's hyponatraemia is a combination of poor dietary intake leading to a relatively low osmolar generation and a thiazide-induced urinary diluting defect (**196**). Final dilution of the urine is dependent on sodium reabsorption by the Na^+/Cl^- transporter in the distal collecting tubule; thiazides inhibit this transporter. The mild urinary diluting defect combined with low osmolar intake predisposes patients to hyponatraemia. SIADH cannot be totally excluded in this patient, but the relatively high uric acid is not consistent with this diagnosis. Psychogenic polydipsia should have a maximally dilute urine.

ii. (a), (b) Fluid restriction and discontinuing the thiazide diurectic should be sufficient in this patient. In general, the serum Na^+ concentration should not be increased by more than 12 mmol during the first 24 hours to avoid the risk of central pontine myelinosis.

197 This radiograph (197) and the blood results given (Table) are from the same patient.
i. What does this IVP show?
ii. What is the explanation for the blood results?

Test	Result
Arterial pH	7.24
[Na$^+$]	136 mmol/l
[Cl$^-$]	110 mmol/l
[HCO$_3^-$]	14 mmol/l

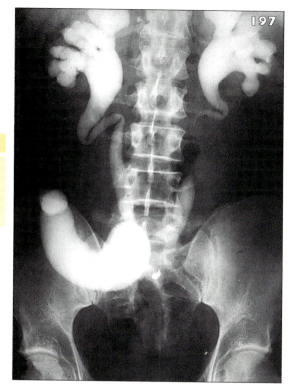

198 Match the most likely aetiology of hyponatraemia with the level of total body sodium (increased, normal or decreased) expected in these conditions:
i. Hypothyroidism.
ii. Adrenal insufficiency.
iii. Syndrome of inappropriate ADH.
iv. Diarrhoea.
v. Congestive heart failure.
vi. Chronic renal failure.
vii. Nausea, pain.

197 i. The IVP shows an ileal conduit.
ii. The blood results show evidence of a normal anion-gap acidosis (anion gap = 12; see 19).

198 Hyponatraemia may be associated with an increase, a decrease or a normal total body sodium volume (Table and see 115).
(a) *Hyponatraemia with decreased total body sodium:* In severe volume depletion, intracellular volume receptors are stimulated, resulting in ADH release which overrides the osmotic stimulus to suppress ADH release. In the presence of diarrhoea or vomiting, urinary Na^+ exretion is low (<10 mEq/l), as the kidney attempts to compensate for sodium losses. In contrast, when sodium is lost through the kidney, urinary sodium excretion is increased (>20 mEq/l).
(b) *Hyponatraemia associated with normal total body volume:* These conditions are associated with either increased ADH levels or increased sensitivity to ADH. Isolated glucocorticoid deficiency is associated with impaired free water excretion, and it has been proposed that glucocorticoids contribute to the normal suppression of ADH. Many drugs can cause hyponatraemia, either by stimulating ADH release or increasing the kidney's sensitivity to ADH. The syndrome of inappropriate ADH (SIADH) is a diagnosis of exclusion and is commonly associated with malignancies (i.e., lung, breast, duodenal, pancreatic, etc) (urinary Na >20 mEq/l).
(c) *Hyponatraemia with increased total body volume:* In cirrhosis, nephrosis and congestive heart failure (CHF), the effective circulating blood volume is decreased which leads to a volume-mediated ADH release. Total body sodium is increased as the kidney attempts to restore intravascular volume (urinary Na^+ <10 mEq/l).

Hyponatraemia		
Decreased total body sodium	**Euvolaemia**	**Increased total body sodium**
Adrenal insufficiency (increased urinary Na^+)	Hypothyroidism	Nephrotic syndrome
Diuretic use (increased urinary Na^+)	Glucocorticoid deficiency	Congestive heart failure
Salt-losing nephritis (increased urinary Na^+)	Syndrome of inappropriate ADH	Hepatic cirrhosis
Osmotic diuresis (increased urinary Na^+)	Pain, nausea	Chronic renal failure (urinary Na^+ variable)
Diarrhoea (decreased urinary Na^+)	Medications	–
Vomiting (decreased urinary Na^+)	–	–

199 This investigation was undertaken in a 14-year-old girl with a history of two urinary tract infections at the age of 2 years who now presents with hypertension.
i. What is the investigation (**199**)?
ii. What does it show?
iii. What is the likely diagnosis?
iv. What is the pathogenesis of these abnormalities?

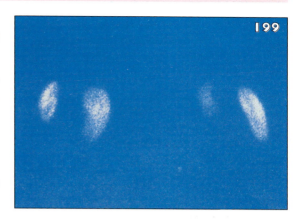

200 This 37-year-old man with a long history of end-stage renal failure developed swelling of his arm (**200**) shortly after the surgical creation of a right brachiocephalic arteriovenous fistula.
i. What is the likely cause of this complication?
ii. What treatment options are available?

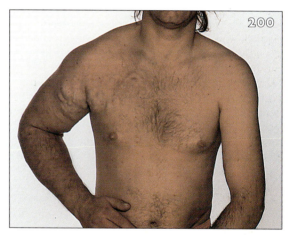

201 This 47-year-old man with juvenile onset diabetes mellitus was doing well until 15 years after renal transplantation when he was noted to have a gradual rise in serum creatinine and proteinuria. Based on this renal biopsy (**201**), what is the most likely cause of his worsening renal function?

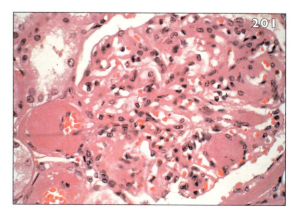

199 i. This is a DMSA (dimercaptosuccinic acid) scan. DMSA binds to tubular cells and therefore images viable renal parenchyma.

ii. This scan shows asymmetrical kidneys with focal indentation of the cortical contour and photon-deficient cortical areas.

iii. The likely diagnosis is chronic pyelonephritis and/or reflux nephropathy.

iv. Acquired segmental scars are thought to be the result of intrarenal reflux of infected urine. Intrarenal reflux does not necessarily occur in all renal papillae. Some papillae, particularly those at the poles of the kidney, tend to be fused structures susceptible to reflux, explaining the polar distribution of segmental scars. However, sustained reflux with an abnormally high bladder pressure can flatten the area cribrosa of an initially non-refluxing papilla, allowing it to reflux. The calyceal clubbing seen on IVP adjacent to cortical scars is the result of papillary distortion and subsequent retraction. Recently it has been suggested that reflux nephropathy may also involve an element of congenital renal dysplasia.

200 i. This man has chronic venous hypertension resulting in the development of a 'brawny arm'. This complication suggests an underlying subclavian vein stenosis or thrombosis. Cannulation of the subclavian vein for haemodialysis vascular access has been popular for almost 20 years. The incidence of subclavian vein stenosis correlates with the duration of catheterisation, and has been reported as a late complication in up to 50% of patients. Such stenoses are usually clinically silent until an ipsilateral arteriovenous fistula (AVF) is fashioned, further elevating venous pressure and resulting in oedema of the upper extremity. Arm swelling can occur immediately after fistula creation or present some months later, often accompanied by clinically obvious venous collaterals (note the venous varicosities over the upper praecordium in this example). In contrast, venous stenosis after internal jugular cannulation is rare, making this the preferred access route.

ii. Anticoagulation with heparin, followed by warfarin, is rarely successful in improving oedema when subclavian vein thrombosis is present. Significant stenosis is sometimes amenable to percutaneous transluminal angioplasty, as the lesion tends to be difficult to approach surgically. Unfortunately, stenosis recurs frequently, necessitating repeat angioplasty or the placement of an intravascular stent. Inoperable stenotic lesions require ligation of the AVF to reduce the oedema.

201 This biopsy reveals the classic changes seen in diabetic nephropathy, including arteriolar hyalinosis, mesangial matrix expansion and a Kimmelstiel–Wilson nodule. Renal histopathological changes characteristic of diabetes mellitus occur with regularity after renal transplantation, although they are usually less severe than those demonstrated here. Clinically significant allograft dysfunction resulting from diabetes is unusual during the first decade following transplantation, and diabetic nephropathy rarely causes allograft failure. Nevertheless, as medical advances lead to longer allograft survival, the incidence of graft failure from recurrent diabetic nephropathy is likely to increase.

202 Shown (202) is the centrifuged urine sediment from an asymptomatic 35-year-old man, viewed with routine light microscopy.
i. What is this finding?
ii. What is its composition?
iii. Under which circumstances might this be found in the urine?

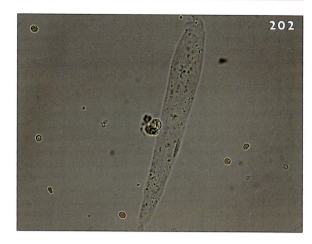

203 A 62-year-old man with recurrent calcium oxalate nephrolithiasis is referred. He has a history of inflammatory bowel disease and coronary artery disease, but no family history of nephrolithiasis. His medications include topical nitroglycerin and oral beta-blockers, and he does not take vitamin D, calcium supplements or diuretics. His physical examination is only notable for mild obesity. Serum laboratory studies include creatinine 1.4 mg/dl (123 µmol/l), bicarbonate 24 mmol/l, calcium 9.6 mg/dl (2.4 mmol/l), phosphorus 3.6 mg/dl (1.2 mmol/l), uric acid 8.1 mg/dl (482 µmol/l) and cholesterol 288 mg/dl (7.4 mmol/l). The results of two 24-hour urine collections, obtained while eating his usual diet, and one urine collection following one week of a low sodium, low calcium, low protein and low oxalate diet are given (Table).
i. What metabolic abnormalities contribute to his nephrolithiasis?
ii. What additional diagnostic test could be useful to confirm the diagnosis?
iii. What therapy should be prescribed?

Test	Usual diet	Usual diet	Low Ca++ diet	Units	Reference values
Volume	1820	2300	1860	ml	–
pH	6	6	6	–	–
Calcium	420	475	140	mg/day	<250 mg/day (males)
Phosphorus	1440	1770	840	mg/day	–
Uric acid	300	460	100	mg/day	<750 mg/day
Creatinine	1700	1850	1500	mg/day	–
Sodium	244	380	117	mmol/day	–
Magnesium	6	6.5	7	mEq/day	>5 mEq/day
Oxalate	36	55	40	mg/day	<40 mg/day
Citrate	24	55	0	mg/day	>250 mg/day

202 i. This is a hyaline cast.

ii. Hyaline casts are formed from Tamm–Horsfall glycoprotein, which is secreted by the ascending limb of the loop of Henle and the distal tubular cells.

iii. Small numbers of hyaline casts are found in the urine of normal individuals. Tamm–Horsfall protein forms casts, particularly in acid pH and when the urine is highly concentrated. Accordingly, casts disappear in dilute, alkaline urine. Hyaline cast formation increases during fever, after strenuous exercise and after the ingestion of thiazide or loop diuretics.

The hyaline cast provides the 'building block' within which all other types of urinary cast are generated. The presence of particulate matter (such as erythrocytes, leucocytes, tubular cells, free fat particles and crystals) within the renal tubular lumen at the time of 'gelling' of the Tamm–Horsfall protein leads to the formation of a pathological urinary cast.

203 i. He has calcium oxalate nephrolithiasis related in part to hypocitruria, hyperoxaluria and hypercalciuria. Urinary citrate is an inhibitor of stone formation, complexing with calcium and decreasing the calcium available to precipitate with other anions. Hyperoxaluria occurs when there is excessive dietary ingestion, increased gastrointestinal absorption or overproduction of oxalate. Hypercalciuria is the most common metabolic abnormality contributing to nephrolithiasis and results from increased intestinal absorption, renal excretion or bone resorption.

ii. Since the patient's urinary calcium excretion normalised in response to a low-sodium, low-calcium diet, his hypercalciuria is due either to absorptive hypercalciuria or excessive dietary sodium intake, which can be differentiated by performing a calcium load test. The patient follows a low-calcium, low-sodium, low-protein and low-oxalate diet for 7 days and then collects a 2-hour urine specimen following a 12-hour fast. After the first 2-hour urine collection he takes a 1 g calcium meal, followed by two consecutive 2-hour urine collections. If the urinary calcium:creatinine ratio is >0.13 before the calcium meal the patient has fasting hypercalciuria. In contrast, if the fasting calcium:creatinine ration is <0.13, but following the calcium mean increases to >0.2, then the patient has absorptive hypercalciuria. Since this patient had a low fasting and low post-absorptive calcium:creatinine ratio, his hypercalciuria is secondary to excessive dietary sodium intake.

iii. Recommendations include both pharmacological and non-pharmacological therapies. He should maintain a high urine output (>2 l/day), restrict dietary sodium (about 2 g/day) and limit dietary oxalate intake. He should also be prescribed potassium citrate, 10–20 mEq three times a day. After 4–6 weeks a repeat 24-hour urine collection is needed to determine if the therapeutic interventions have been successful. If his urine oxalate remains high and he is able to maintain a low salt diet, calcium carbonate should be prescribed to bind intestinal oxalate.

204 A 20-year-old student is found to have a blood pressure of 242/134 mmHg in physiology class. Her hands are shown in **204a**.

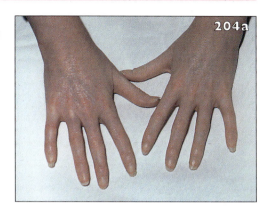

i. What abnormalities can you see?
ii. What other features in the history or examination would assist you in making a diagnosis?
iii. The kidney is affected by this condition – what are the histological features?
iv. How would you manage this patient?

205 A 12-year-old girl with spina bifida is referred for evaluation and management. Unfortunately, her urinary incontinence has been managed by wearing a diaper. A renal ultrasound reveals bilateral hydronephrosis. A VCUG is performed (**205**).

i. What does the VCUG show?
ii. What is the appropriate management?

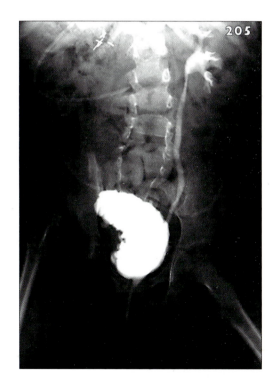

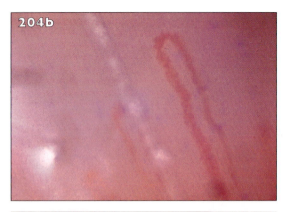

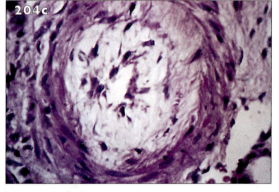

204 i. There is tightness of the skin over the fingers with 'pinching' of the finger ends consistent with systemic sclerosis.

ii. In the history, oesophageal involvement may be associated with dysphagia. Patients may also complain of a change in their facial appearance, tightness of the perioral skin and Raynaud's phenomenon. Calcinosis and telangectasia of the fingers may also be seen on examination. Capillaroscopy may assist by showing dilatation of the nail fold capillaries (**204b**).

iii. Renal biopsy (**204c**) in systemic sclerosis shows intimal hyperplasia and fibrous thickening of the adventita and perivascular tissues of the intralobular and arcuate arteries, which is associated with ischaemic glomerulosclerosis.

iv. Optimal control of blood pressure should be the priority in managing this patient. Penicillamine can be used in an attempt to decrease tissue fibrosis, but its efficacy is limited.

205 i. The VCUG reveals an enlarged, trabeculated bladder and left-sided vesicoureteral reflux.

ii. As part of this patient's evaluation a urine culture should be performed to exclude a urinary tract infection. Video urodynamics should also be performed to measure intravesicular pressure and to evaluate the bladder anatomy associated with this neurogenic condition. Treatment is directed at facilitating bladder emptying and decreasing the intravesicular pressure. Options include intermittent self-catheterisation, oral anticholinergics, urinary diversion and augmentation cystoplasty.

206 An elderly man with a 4-year history of Type II NIDDM is referred because of renal insufficiency. Blood pressure is 158/94 mmHg and physical examination is normal except for leg oedema. Serum creatinine is 2.2 mg/dl (195 µmol/l), albumin 35 g/l, cholesterol 267 mg/dl (6.9 mmol/l) and haemoglobin A1c 11%. Urinalysis reveals 4+ protein, 1+ blood, 1+

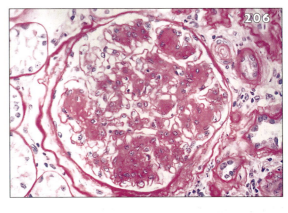

glucose, 5–8 RBCs HPF and 2+ granular casts. Proteinuria is 3.5 g/day and creatinine clearance 56 ml/min. By ultrasound, the kidneys are 12 cm in length, without masses or hydronephrosis. Serum protein electrophoresis shows no monoclonal spike and urine electrophoresis is negative for Bence Jones proteins. Fundoscopic examination is normal. A kidney biopsy is performed (**206**, courtesy of R. Hennigar, MD).
i. What is the most likely diagnosis?
ii. What therapy is indicated?

207 This 68-year-old man has urine protein of 10.2 g/24 h and a serum albumin of 26 g/l. His face was normal 3 months prior to his appearance in **207**.
i. What are the periorbital lesions?
ii. Why have they developed so rapidly?
iii. Should treatment be considered?
iv. What therapy should be considered?

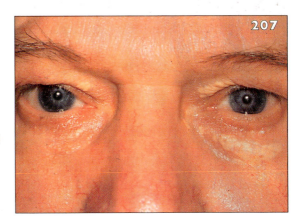

206 i. The biopsy shows a glomerulus with nodular mesangial expansion with minimal hypercellularity, suggestive of diabetic glomerulosclerosis (Kimmelsteil–Wilson nodules). Similar histological findings can be seen in light chain nephropathy, which should excluded by immunofluorescence and electron microscopy (EM) studies. A kidney biopsy was performed in this patient because of the atypical presentation – nephrotic syndrome with renal insufficiency in a patient with a brief history of diabetes and no evidence of diabetic retinopathy.

The natural history of nephropathy in NIDDM is similar to that in IDDM. Renal histology is also identical. However, in contrast to IDDM, microalbuminuria is not a predictor of nephropathy in NIDDM. Whereas more than 90% of IDDM patients with microalbuminuria will progress to overt nephropathy, only 20–30% of microalbuminuric NIDDM patients develop clinical nephropathy. Thus, in NIDDM the diagnosis of diabetic nephropathy can only be made on clinical grounds when *macro*albuminuria (>300 mg/d) is present. In those NIDDM patients with microalbuminuria who do not develop clinical nephropathy, the microalbuminuria is thought to result from vascular rather than glomerular damage. In this population, microalbuminuria is a strong correlate of cardiovascular mortality.

207 i. Xanthelasma.
ii. This man has nephrotic syndrome, a cause of secondary hypercholesterolaemia. Serum cholesterol may be very high [in this case, 483 mg/dl (12.5 mmol/l)] and may rise rapidly so that the cutaneous stigmata of hypercholesterolaemia develop in a short time.
The hyperlipidaemia may be mixed with increased triglyceride; triglyceride particularly rises in severe nephrotic syndrome – serum albumin <20 g/l. The aetiology of hypercholesterolaemia is complex – in addition to impaired LDL clearance, there is overproduction of VLDL which rapidly degrades, resulting in an increased LDL formation. Lipoprotein lipase activity may also be reduced, leading to impaired triglyceride clearance.
iii. It is not the xanthelasma which justify treatment, but the underlying lipid abnormality. Increased cardiovascular morbidity and mortality are a feature of chronic renal disease in general, and of nephrotic syndrome in particular. Hyperlipidaemia is one risk factor which should be modified if possible. However, direct evidence that lipid lowering agents reduce cardiovascular mortality in nephrotics is lacking.
iv. Treatment for the hyperlipidaemia of nephrotic syndrome has been difficult. Diet alone may be inadequate and fibrates and cholestyramine have unacceptable side effects. HMG CoA reductase inhibitors ('statins') have now been shown to be safe and effective. Nevertheless, cholesterol levels recommended for the general population may not be achievable.

208 Shown (**208**, courtesy of Peritoneal Dialysis International) are the results of a peritoneal equilibration test in a patient treated by CAPD. Net ultrafiltration during the test was 620 ml.
i. How is the test performed?
ii. What do the results indicate in this patient?

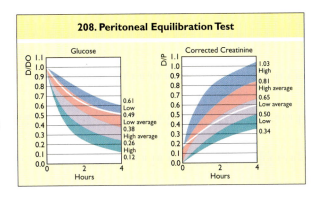

208. Peritoneal Equilibration Test

209 A newborn, full-term baby boy had been followed *in utero* with prenatal ultrasonography for right-sided hydro-ureteronephrosis. To investigate this further a MAG3 renogram is obtained (**209**).
i. What would your differential diagnosis be before the renogram?
ii. What investigation should be undertaken before a renogram?
iii. What does the renogram show?

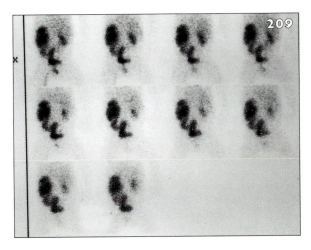

210 A patient underwent treatment for acute rejection on three separate occasions during the first 6 months after transplantation. Shortly thereafter, he developed fevers and night sweats. This chest radiograph (**210**) was obtained. What is the differential diagnosis?

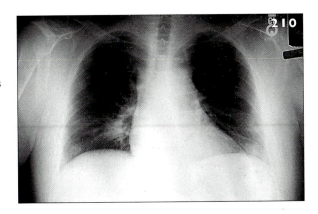

208 i. The test measures ultrafiltration capacity and the equilibration rates of glucose and creatinine using a standard 2 l exchange of 2.27% dextrose over 4 hours. The test provides an index of the peritoneal transport characteristics for a given patient and may be used as a guide to choosing their optimum dialysis prescription. A single plasma creatinine concentration, and dialysate creatinine and glucose concentrations at 2 and 4 hours, in addition to the effluent volume at 4 hours, are measured. Results are expressed as dialysate to plasma creatinine ratios, dialysate glucose at 2 and 4 hours to dialysate glucose at time 0 and net ultrafiltration. Since glucose may interfere with the creatinine assay, plasma and, in particular, dialysate creatinine levels must be corrected for glucose.
ii. This patient has adequate ultrafiltration at 4 hours, below average creatinine equilibration and average glucose absorption. He should be suitable for conventional CAPD, but perhaps using large volume exchanges.

209 i. Three diagnoses should be considered in this infant; right ureteral obstruction, right ureteral reflux and a non-obstructed, non-refluxing megaureter.
ii. A VCUG should be performed to exclude reflux and urethral obstruction.
iii. The MAG3 renogram shows a right-sided megaureter. The decision whether to operate on a patient with asymptomatic hydronephrosis is determined by the level of residual renal function. If renal function is more than 40% of normal, many paediatric urologists would recommend repeating the renogram in 3–6 months.

210 The differential diagnosis for nodular pulmonary infiltrates in an immunosuppressed renal transplant recipient is long. Infectious causes include Mycobacterial infections (especially *Mycobacterium tuberculosis*), *Aspergillus fumigatus*, *Nocardia asteroides*, *Pneumocystis carinii*, *Cryptococcus neoformans*, *Histoplasma capsulatum*, *Coccidioides immitis* and *Blastomyces dermatiditis*. In addition to infectious causes, primary lung and metastatic tumours and Hodgkin's and (less commonly) non-Hodgkin's lymphomas can cause nodular pulmonary infiltrates. Masqueraders not to be forgotten include pulmonary emboli and occasionally focal pulmonary oedema. This patient had a non-Hodgkin's lymphoma.

211 A 35-year-old man presents with progressive renal insufficiency, mild proteinuria and haematuria. His fasting blood sugar is normal, but he does have a family history of diabetes mellitus and premature strokes. Ophthalmological examination to exclude diabetic retinopathy reveals tortuous retinal vessels and concentric, 'onion-skin'-appearing deposits in his cornea. Reddish papules are scattered over his lower trunk and extremities. Which of the following would the renal biopsy show?
i. Longitudinal splitting of GBMs.
ii. Glomerular epithelial 'foam' cells.
iii. Thickening of the TBM.
iv. Moth-eaten appearance of GBM.

212 Patients A (**212a**) and B (**212b**) (courtesy of Mrs V. Broomhead) have both had the same laboratory test.
i. What is the test?
ii. What is the result in the two patients?
iii. What possible diagnoses should be considered?

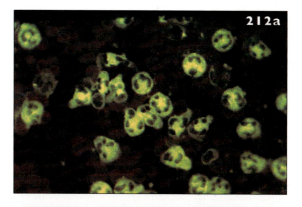

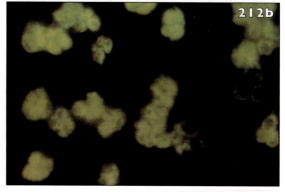

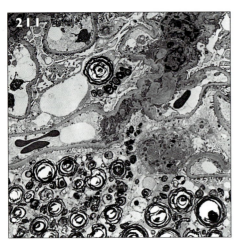

211 ii. Glomerular epithelial 'foam' cells. Fabry's disease (angiokeratoma corporis diffusum universale) is an X-linked recessive disorder due to deficient activity of the lysosomal hydrolase, α-galactosidase A. This defect leads to progressive accumulation of neutral glycosphingolipids, in various tissues, including the kidneys. Renal disease manifests as haematuria, mild proteinuria and progressive renal insufficiency. Examination of renal biopsy material reveals that every cell type shows vacuolisation from the accumulation of glycosphingolipids. On light microscopy, enlarged glomerular epithelial cells with a 'foamy' appearance are filled with multiple small, clear vacuoles. Electron microscopy reveals that these vacuoles consist of round, lamellated structures called 'zebra bodies' (211). ESRD in affected men typically occurs in the fifth decade of life. Initial optimism that renal transplantation would serve as a source of normal enzymes has waned. However, long-term kidney function has been reported following kidney transplantation for Fabry's disease.

Other manifestations of Fabry's disease include cutaneous papular lesions clustered on the lower torso and extremities, acroparesthesias and premature coronary and carotid insufficiency. Tortuous retinal vessels and whorled corneal epithelial deposits are pathognomonic findings. Phenotypically classic men may have no detectable enzyme, a non-functional enzyme or qualitative enzyme defects related to abnormal protein synthesis, stability or processing. In studies of men from unrelated families affected with Fabry's disease, six different gene rearrangements, five partial deletions, one partial duplication and multiple point mutations have been recognised.

212 i. The investigation is an indirect immunofluorescence assay on ethanol-fixed human neutrophils for antibodies to neutrophil cytoplasmic antigen (ANCA).
ii. The result from patient A shows a cytoplasmic pattern (c-ANCA) and patient B a nuclear–perinuclear pattern (p-ANCA). The antigens most commonly associated with c- and p-ANCA are proteinase 3 and myeloperoxidase, respectively, although other antigens can be involved, including lactoferrin, lysozyme, elasatase and cathepsin G.
iii. Wegener's granulomatosis is more frequently associated with c-ANCA (anti-proteinase 3), whereas in microscopic polyarteritis nodosa c- and p-ANCA (anti-myeloperoxidase) are evenly distributed. p-ANCA is found more frequently in idiopathic crescentic glomerulonephritis and Churg–Strauss syndrome.

213 A 19-year-old man with a history of recurrent calcium oxalate nephrolithiasis presents with nausea, malaise and pruritus. He has a normal blood pressure, pale conjunctiva and trace lower extremity oedema. His laboratory studies show creatinine 5.1 mg/dl (451 µmol/l), urea nitrogen 70 mg/dl (25 mmol/l), potassium 5.4 mmol/l, bicarbonate 18 mmol/l, phosphorus 7.0 mg/dl (2.3 mmol/l) and calcium 8.2 mg/dl (2.05 mmol/l). Renal ultrasound reveals normal-sized kidneys with multiple echogenicities consistent with nephrolithiasis but no obstruction. Serological examination was normal and 24-hour protein excretion was 350 mg/day. The renal biopsy is shown in **213**.

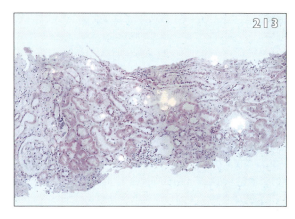

i. What is the aetiology of his renal failure.

ii. What is the treatment?

214 A 30-year-old man is found semiconscious on the floor of his room by friends. He is taken to the local emergency room, where he complains of general malaise and pain in his right leg and shoulder. His friends give a history of alcohol abuse. On examination there is bruising and swelling of the lateral aspect of his right thigh and shoulder area. Serum creatinine is 4.5 mg/dl (400 µmol/l), BUN 42 mg/dl (15 mmol/l) and creatine kinase 40,000 IU/ml. Urinalysis shows protein 3+ and blood 3+; urine microscopy reveals red cells and pigmented casts. A renal biopsy is undertaken (**214**).

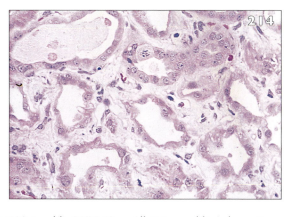

What does the biposy show and what is the probable diagnosis?

213 i. Examination of the renal biopsy with polarised light demonstrated calcium oxalate deposition within the tubules consistent with primary hyperoxaluria. Primary hyperoxaluria is an autosomal recessive defect in one of two enzymes that results in overproduction of oxalate. Type 1 primary hyperoxaluria is the most common and results from a deficiency in hepatic alanine:glyoxalate aminotransferase (AGT). Type 2 primary hyperoxaluria results from a defect in cytosolic glyoxalate reductase/D-glycerate dehydrogenase. These patients form calcium oxalate stones at an early age and can progress to chronic renal failure. As renal failure progresses, excretion of oxalate decreases and calcium oxalate precipitates in tissues (systemic oxalosis). This results in cardiac conduction defects, digit necrosis, synovitis and pathological fractures.

ii. Patients with primary hyperoxaluria should maintain high urine outputs (>3 l/day) and avoid oxalate-rich foods. Some patients with Type 1 primary hyperoxaluria respond to high-dose pyridoxine (a coenzyme for AGT). Oral citrates may be of benefit by increasing the calcium oxalate solubility. Once renal failure develops, patients with Type 1 primary hyperoxaluria should be considered for combined liver–kidney transplant, since isolated kidney transplant is of minimal benefit because of the high incidence of recurrent disease.

214 The biopsy shows acute tubular necrosis. The probable diagnosis is rhabdomyolysis, which is predisposed by alcohol consumption. Myoglobulin, which is directly nephrotoxic, can sometime be found in the urine, but its absence does not rule out the diagnosis. Serum creatinine is often higher than expected from renal impairment alone; this is due to direct release of creatinine with muscle breakdown. Creatine kinase levels are markedly elevated. Ionised calcium concentration is often low on presentation, due to muscle binding; hypercalcaemia can be a feature of the recovery phase. In most cases the prognosis for recovery of renal function is good.

215 You are asked to see an 8-year-old child in paediatric renal clinic. The youngster's father explains that the family recently emigrated from Nigeria, and that his son has been lethargic, with intermittent fevers and chills for several weeks. He also states that his son's abdomen has become distended and that his legs are swollen. Physical examination reveals periorbital oedema, ascites with a palpable spleen and 3+ pitting ankle oedema. Urine shows 3+ protein, 2+ blood and no glucose. The urinary sediment is shown in **215a** and **215b** (courtesy Arthur Greenberg).

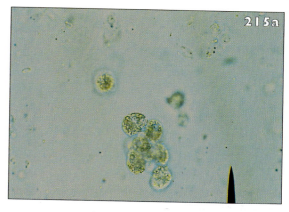
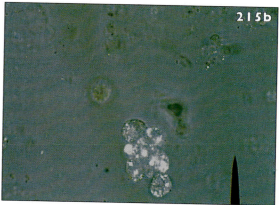

i. What is your differential diagnosis?
ii. Which disease is most likely and how would you confirm the diagnosis?

216 A 59-year-old man with a 20-year history of gout is referred for evaluation of renal insufficiency. His medications include colchicine and intermittent NSAID use. He has no occupational or social exposure to lead. His blood pressure is normal and his examination reveals the abnormality shown (**216**). Serum chemistries reveal a creatinine of 2.2 mg/dl (195 μmol/l), potassium 4.1 mmol/l, total CO_2 23 mmol/l and uric acid 11 mg/dl (654 μmol/l). His urinalysis and serologic evaluations were normal.

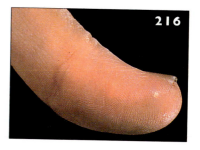

i. What is the aetiology of his renal disease?
ii. What therapy should be prescribed?

215 i. The urinary sediment in (215a) shows an oval fat body which, when viewed under polarised light, demonstrates 'Maltese crosses' (215b). This finding is strongly suggestive of nephrotic-range proteinuria. In the United States, minimal change disease (MCD) is the most common cause of childhood nephrotic syndrome, accounting for 80–95% of the cases in children 1–6 years of age. In older children the incidence of MCD declines to about 65%. Several features of this case make MCD less likely – haematuria is rare in minimal change disease and persistent episodic fever and chills are also unusual. These findings, combined with the child's country of origin, must raise the issue of nephrotic syndrome secondary to malaria.

ii. The diagnosis could be confirmed by renal biopsy. Malaria due to *Plasmodium falciparum* is frequently associated with proteinuria (about 50%), but less than 1% develop nephrotic syndrome. The most common histological lesion seen is MPGN (MCGN) (35% in one study). Focal GN and membranous glomerular changes accounted for 14% and 12%, respectively; and 22% had minimal change disease. In these patients treatment with antimalarial drugs is usually associated with renal functional improvement over 1–2 months.

Infection with *Plasmodium malariae* (quartan malaria) is associated with one-third of the cases of nephrotic syndrome in Uganda and Nigeria, where the disease is endemic. Thickening of the glomerular capillary wall with double contours of the GBM on silver stain is characteristic of renal damage due to *P. malariae* and has been dubbed 'quartan malarial nephropathy'. It is thought to occur due to the deposition of antigen–antibody complexes in the glomerulus. Prognosis is poor and the disease tends to progress despite therapy with antimalarial drugs, corticosteroids and cytotoxic drugs.

216 i. 216 reveals a tophi in his distal phalanx, suggesting the possibility of chronic urate nephropathy. Urate nephropathy occurs in the setting of severe tophaceous gout and hyperuricaemia. It is the result of chronic uric acid deposition in the medullary interstitium leading to an inflammatory response and interstitial nephritis. There may be a history of lead exposure. An additional confounding variable in many cases of urate nephropathy and chronic renal failure is the long-standing use of NSAIDs.

ii. Treatment is directed at lowering the serum uric acid level and reabsorption of the tophi. Uricosuric agents are of limited use in this patient because they are ineffective in the presence of renal insufficiency. Therefore, the drug of choice is allopurinol. Finally, general measures to slow the progression of renal failure, such as strict blood pressure control and low-protein diets, may be considered.

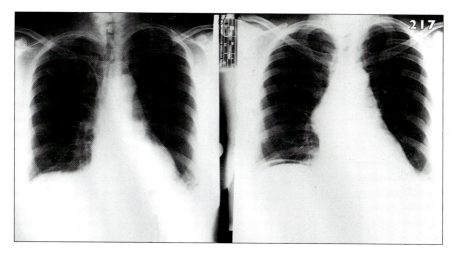

217 A 49-year-old woman presented with end-stage renal failure. A percutaneous subclavian haemodialysis catheter was positioned uneventfully using the infraclavicular approach under local anaesthesia. The check chest radiograph demonstrated good catheter position, with no apparent complications from the insertion procedure (217, left panel). Shortly after the commencement of haemodialysis, the patient complained of severe central chest pain. She remained haemodynamically stable, but dialysis was discontinued. A repeat radiograph explained her symptoms, her dialysis catheter was removed, and she was converted to peritoneal dialysis. Explain the changes demonstrated on her later radiograph (217, right panel).

218 This CAPD patient (218) complains of thirst and increasing shortness of breath.
i. What is the diagnosis?
ii. What treatment should be advised?

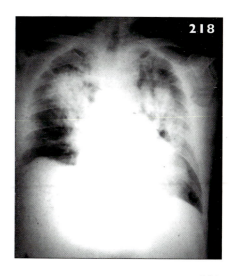

217 The patient's chest pain was caused by an acute haemomediastinum following subclavian cannulation for haemodialysis. Subclavian catheters provide reliable temporary vascular access for haemodialysis, but serious complications may occur during, or shortly after, the insertion procedure, particularly if performed by an inexperienced operator. Inadvertent puncture of nearby structures may lead to pneumothorax, subclavian artery haemorrhage, brachial plexus injury and thoracic duct laceration. The literature also contains reports of the trachea and the carotid and vertebral arteries being punctured during the attempted placement of a subclavian catheter. Fatal air embolus may also occur.

Perforation of the vasculature, during subclavian vein cannulation may result in life-threatening complications, such as haemothorax or pericardial tamponade (see **176**). In this example chest pain was caused by the expanding mediastinal haematoma (confirmed by CT), exacerbated by the anticoagulation of the dialysis procedure. The haematoma is clearly seen as a 'bulge' along the right margin of the mediastinum. [The air present under the right hemidiaphragm (right panel) was the consequence of the subsequent insertion of a peritoneal dialysis catheter].

218 i. The chest radiograph (**218**) shows cardiomegaly and pulmonary oedema. Increased thirst is common in patients receiving peritoneal dialysis, and may be exacerbated by the use of hypertonic exchanges. In the absence of generalised volume overload, causes of poor left ventricular function, such as a recent myocardial infarction, should be excluded.

ii. The patient with generalised volume overload may have ultrafiltration failure, but excessive fluid intake is more likely. A careful history, supported if necessary by measuring ultrafiltration capacity when the patient is euvolaemic, will establish the aetiology. Patient education regarding limiting both fluid intake and the use of hypertonic exchanges may help prevent recurrence. In patients with ultrafiltration failure a change to haemodialysis should be considered.

219 A young woman with a 12-year history of Type I IDDM is referred because of progressive pedal oedema. On examination, she is normotensive, without signs of heart failure or liver disease. Pedal oedema is present. Serum chemistries are normal, except for an albumin of 34 g/l. Urinalysis shows 3+ protein, but is negative for blood, glucose and ketones; urinary

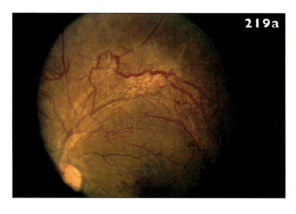

sediment is bland. Proteinuria is quantitated at 2.6 g/day with a creatinine clearance of 112 ml/min. Funduscopic examination is shown (219a, courtesy of A. Capone, MD).
i. What is the most likely diagnosis?
ii. What therapy is indicated?

220 A 25-year-old woman developed severe hypertension in pregnancy. This persisted after delivery and she was referred for investigation. A renal arteriogram was undertaken (220).
i. What does the arteriogram show?
ii. Might this condition have been diagnosed in any other way?
iii. What treatment should be recommended?

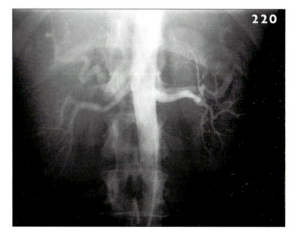

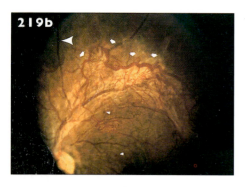

219 i. The most likely diagnosis is diabetic nephropathy. 219b (courtesy of A. Capone, MD) shows proliferative diabetic retinopathy with microaneuryms (small arrowheads), and a large neovascular trunk vessel with fine arborizing neovascularisation (arrows). The large arrowhead points to a normal retinal vein. The diagnosis of diabetic nephropathy is usually based on clinical criteria; kidney biopsy is reserved for cases with atypical features. The criteria for the diagnosis of diabetic nephropathy include:

- Temporal course compatible with the natural history of diabetic renal disease.
- Additional evidence of organ damage from diabetes, e.g., diabetic retinopathy or neuropathy.
- 'Bland' urinary sediment and negative serological evaluation for other causes of proteinuria.

Approximately 30% of patients with Type I diabetes will eventually develop renal failure. Of patients with diabetic nephropathy 90% will also have diabetic retinopathy. The absence of retinopathy in a patient being evaluated for diabetic nephropathy should cast doubt on the diagnosis, and prompt further evaluation.

ii. Besides optimising glycaemic control, treatment should be directed at reducing proteinuria, slowing the rate of progression of renal failure and correcting hyperlipidaemia. Strict blood pressure control has been shown to reduce proteinuria and to slow the rate of progression of renal failure. Recently, the converting enzyme inhibitor captopril has been shown to have a therapeutic advantage in slowing progressive diabetic renal failure compared with other antihypertensives, despite similar systemic blood pressure control. Moderate protein restriction (0.6–0.7 g/kg/day) may also reduce proteinuria and the rate of progression of diabetic nephropathy. Hyperlipidaemia should also be treated to reduce cardiovascular mortality.

220 i. The arteriogram (220) shows fibromuscular dysplasia, a condition that most commonly affects the renal arteries, but other arteries may be involved.
ii. Renal angiography with direct intra-arterial injection is the gold standard for the diagnosis of renal artery stenosis. The images obtained with digital subtraction angiography lack the clarity necessary for diagnosis, duplex Doppler ultrasound is operator-dependent and MRI and spiral CT angiography are at present being assessed.
iii. Angioplasty is the treatment of choice in fibromuscular dysplasia. Two-thirds of patients are cured and the remainder show a significant improvement in hypertensive control. In contrast, atheromatous renal artery stenosis is associated with a less than 20% cure rate.

Abbreviations

ABG, arterial blood gas
ACE, angiotensin-converting enzyme
ACEI, angiotensin-converting enzyme inhibitor
ACKD, acquired cystic kidney disease
ADH, antidiuretic hormone
ADPKD, autosomal dominant polycystic kidney disease
AER, albumin excretion rate
AFB, acid-fast bacillus
AGT, alanine:glyoxalate aminotransferase
AIDS, acquired immunodeficiency syndrome
AIN, allergic interstitial nephritis
AL, immunoglobulin light chains
ALT, alanine aminotransferase
AMA, arm muscle area
AMC, arm muscle circumference
ANCA, anti-neutrophil cytoplasmic antibodies
ARF, acute renal failure
ARPKD, autosomal recessive polycystic kidney disease
ASD, atrial septal defect
AST, aspartate aminotransferase
ATN, acute tubular necrosis
AV, arteriovenous
AVF, arteriovenous fistula
B2M, beta2-microglobulin
BRCN, bilateral renal cortical necrosis
BUN, blood urea nitrogen
C3Nef, C3 nephritic factor
CAPD, continuous ambulatory peritoneal dialysis
CAVH, continuous arteriovenous haemofiltration
CAVHD, continuous arteriovenous haemodialysis
CCT, cortical collecting tubule
CCU, critical care unit
CHF, congestive heart failure
CMV, cytomegalovirus
CNS, central nervous system
CRF, chronic renal failure

CPK, creatine phosphokinase
CSA, cyclosporin
CT, computerised tomography
CVA, costovertebral angle
CVP, central venous pressure
CVVH, continuous venovenous haemofiltration
CVVHD, continuous venovenous haemodialysis
DMSA, dimercaptosuccinic acid
EBV, Ebstein–Barr virus
ECG, electrocardiagram
EM, electron microscopy
ESR, erythrocyte sedimentation rate
ESRD, end-stage renal disease
ESWL, Extracorporeal shock-wave lithotripsy
ETO, ethylene oxide
FMF, Familial Mediterranean fever
FSGS, focal segmental glomerulosclerosis
GBM, glomerular basement membrane
GFR, glomerular filtration rate
GN, glomerulonephritis
HDL, High density lipoprotein
HELLP, haemolysis, elevated liver enzymes and low platelets
Hgb, haemoglobins
HIV, human immunodeficiency virus
HMG-CoA, 3-hydroxy-3-methylglutaryl coenzyme A
HPF, high power field
HPLC, high performance liquid chromatography
HPV, human papillomavirus
HSP, Henoch–Schönlein purpura
HUS, haemolytic uraemic syndrome
IGF, insulin-like growth factor
IDDM, insulin dependent diabetes mellitus
JVP, jugular venous pressure
IVP, intravenous pyelogram (also known as intravenous urogram, IVU)
KUB, kidney, ureter and bladder
LDL, low density lipoprotein

Abbreviations

MAC, mid-arm circumference
MCD, minimal change disease
MCGN, mesangiocapillary glomeru-
lonephritis
MCT, medullary collecting tubule
MEN II, multiple endocrine neoplasia
syndrome Type II
MIBG, metaiodobenzylguanidine
MIDD, monoclonal immunoglobulin
deposition diseases
MPGN, membranoproliferative
glomerulonephritis
MRI, magnetic resonance imaging
NIDDM, non-insulin dependent dia-
betes mellitus
NSAIDs, non-steroidal anti-inflammato-
ry drugs
PFD, paired filtration dialysis
PT, prothrombin time
PTH, parathyroid hormone
PTT, partial thromboplastin time
RA, rheumatoid arthritis

RBC, red blood cell
RTA, renal tubular acidosis
SBE, subacute bacterial endocarditis
SGA, subjective global assessment
SIADH, syndrome of inappropriate
ADH
SLE, systemic lupus erythematosus
SSA, serum amyloid A
TALH, thick ascending limb of Henle
TBM, tubular basement membrane
TGF, tumour growth factor
TTKG, transtubular potassium gradient
TURP, transurethral resection of
prostate
UKM, urea kinetic modelling
UTI, urinary tract infection
VCUG, voiding cystourethrogram
VLDL, very low density lipoprotein
VURD, valves, unilateral reflux and dys-
plasia
WBC, white blood cell

Index

Index

Index

Index